# The Teachings of Dora Kalff
*Sandplay*

Published by

TEMENOS PRESS®
Box 305
Cloverdale, California 95425
USA
www.temenospress.com

ISBN 978-0-9728517-9-4

First Edition
*With thanks to Bonnie Wilkins for graphics assistance*

**Library of Congress Cataloging-in-Publication Data**

The teachings of Dora Kalff : sandplay / Barbara A. Turner,
   editor. -- 1st ed.

   p. cm.
   Includes bibliographical references and index.
   LCCN 2013932124
   ISBN 978-0-9728517-9-4

   1. Sandplay--Therapeutic use.  2. Play therapy.
   3. Jungian psychology.   I. Kalff, Dora M.  II. Turner,
   Barbara A.

   RC489.S25T43 2013      616.89'1653
                          QBI13-600021

*For my students in sandplay*
*who carry on the work of*
*Dora Kalff*

# Table of Contents

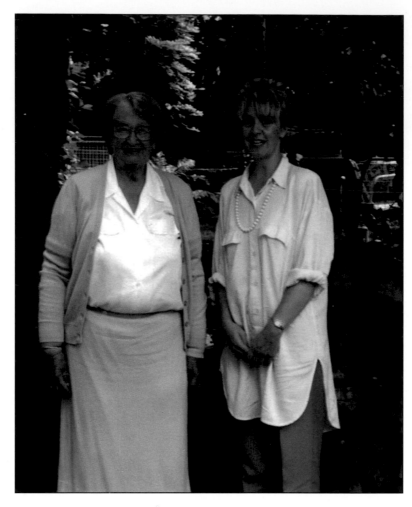

**Dora Kalff and Barbara Turner, 1988, Zollikon, Switzerland**

# The Teachings of Dora Kalff
## Sandplay®

### *Preface*

What follows are the teachings of Dora Kalff transcribed from the notes I made at the time in shorthand. We cannot assume that they are as complete as would be a voice recording, however we can "hear" her voice in her words. I feel that these are treasures in the history of sandplay® and want to share them with others, particularly those who did not have the opportunity to study directly with this remarkable teacher.

I have done my best to leave her language as she spoke it, and have made only minor edits for purposes of continuity and understanding. A few items requiring definition are added and enclosed in parentheses. I have also included some additional materials elaborating on some of the references Mrs. Kalff makes in her lectures. Gender references have been left as they were spoken. In many cases the masculine referent is used, as was the custom at the time. For purposes of privacy and confidentiality all identifying information has been removed from the cases. The clients are spoken about in respectful, but general terms. The sandplays are replications I constructed from the sketches I drew of the photos and the verbal descriptions Mrs. Kalff gave during her lectures. In many cases it was necessary to make the figures she described, as they are no longer commonly available. The drawings are similarly reproduced from my notes made during the seminars. We can assume that the trays and drawings look very unlike their originals, but they do provide us with a visual example of what she spoke about. An index is included to facilitate study and research, as is a list of references mentioned in the text, and resources for training in sandplay.

It was an honor to have studied with Dora Kalff. I first met her at the lectures she gave in Northern California in 1987. We were so fortunate then, because she would visit the area and do several workshops and talks about sandplay. She was a rather quiet and small woman, but her presence filled every available space in a room. Wherever she went, large crowds hushed to listen to what she had to say.

Dora Kalff spoke with deep conviction about the Self, the center of the personality, as the birthright of every human being. She clarified that recovering and developing the Self was the core of our work in psychotherapy. The audiences were riveted and inspired by the clarity of her perceptions, which stemmed from a profound understanding of what is true. She told us that this work is demanding, that not everyone can do it, and that it requires our own personal development and humility. Humbly holding the work was central for Mrs. Kalff. She would not tolerate any inflated egos around sandplay. When someone began saying how many sand trays they saw each week, or the great ambitions they had with sandplay, she would swiftly knock them off of their pedestals. Above all, Dora Kalff unreservedly affirmed that there was simply nothing more important than *our* continued task to align with the Self.

I was very fortunate to do the three-week study program with Dora Kalff at her home in Zollikon, Switzerland, in 1988. My work in sandplay deepened profoundly and these studies awakened even more questions in me about how sandplay works to move the psyche. In addition, my personal sandplay work with Mrs. Kalff gave me direction for the balance of my professional career. I am so grateful for the gift of this amazing teacher in my life. I have the deepest respect for her and hope that you will enjoy sharing some of her wisdom.

*Barbara A. Turner, PhD*
*Cloverdale, California*
*January 2013*

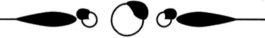

# Sandplay with Adolescents

*4th – 6th March 1988*

Sandplay is about play. Play has to do with spontaneity and not thinking. There is concentration. The child moves from an object to a subject. For example, the doll becomes a baby. Schiller said man is only human when he plays. Play is the capacity to express freely with inner motivation. This motivation comes from the Self, the total aspect of the human being – both conscious and unconscious.

We are born with this totality. This is like a seed, the Self. There is much potential in this seed which is ready to be developed. During the first year of life, the Self is contained completely in the mother's life. As soon as the child stands and walks, he alienates from the mother. The Self begins to move out. Between two and four years, the Self is manifested in the child. The child begins to draw circles and squares. Pay attention to what the child expresses at this age and what questions come up at this age. They begin to ask about God. At this moment they are near the Self. These are archetypal expressions, common all over the world. We are born with it. We have access to our potentials and can transcend to divine qualities.

Today we forget about these things that we received by birth. We look out instead of inward.

When the child is able to manifest the Self, the blooming begins. A healthy ego can be developed. The ego is under the guidance of the Self. The ego is in constant connection with this total aspect that is given at birth.

When it is impossible for the child to manifest this possibility, it becomes what Neumann calls a *"needy ego."* The needy ego is insecure. It can become aggressive or depressive. It can also develop to some extent quite well. People can live with it until some misfortune happens. At puberty we see children who cannot learn certain things, even though they have high IQ's. These are the children we see in practice. We should give them the chance to be perfect. To do this we need knowledge of the Self, of these inner qualities that have been left aside.

It is hard to ask the child about dreams. Sandplay can fulfill this task. Sandplay is a path toward the deeper layers within us.

At the beginning in sandplay, we observe images of the daily world, its difficulties. When we continue this work, we get into deeper realms of ourselves. We discover contents which have remained unknown. They have become dark and negative. All of our potentials would like to be developed. If they are not taken care of, they get furious and work against us.

Beyond this darkness is the beauty of the Self. This is a moment when a transformation of energy can take place, because the moment is in tune with the transpersonal qualities within us. This is no longer just personal, but it is universal. From here we build up a new personality, where the ego is in contact with the Self. It is guided by the Self. We can make use of more and greater capacities than before.

This person can be happier, less jealous. When one can live up to his capacities, he will feel good in himself and will not look jealously at the other person. Sandplay develops this path that is indicated by birth.

Sandplay is not as simple as it seems. People who want to use sandplay as a tool should have undergone sandplay, or a therapeutic path to develop their Self. When we are in tune with ourselves, we have great capacity to feel in balance. We are joyful and are able to concentrate on what is coming from the other. You can take what the other brings. You do not have to criticize or judge. You just accept whatever they bring into the practice.

This will be *contained*. This container is where the whole process of the other can develop freely. You accept and experience what they bring. This facilitates a movement in the other toward the deeper layers of themselves. Jung said that unless you have experienced what you want to be for others, you cannot bring anyone further than you are yourself.

If you can provide a free and protected space, you will see the evolution of life as it is taking place in the sand tray. The figures make the connection from the inner to the outer world. This brings inner contents into the outer reality. The inner reality is real. I do not call it a fantasy. This is a personal reality, as well as a collective reality. When we touch the Self, this is a divine reality.

If we get in connection with the Self, it is always accompanied by a numinous experience. This numinosity is real. It is difficult to describe, but we know when it happens. We no longer feel alone; we feel protected and we see beauty that we have never seen. We see openings to problems. We are grateful beyond expression. We all have the capacity to experience this.

In Japan, transference is not achieved by talking. They talk about the *hara* (gut) transference. It is a power, or energy. They do not need to talk to understand each other. They understand what it is to *be* together.

In puberty we leave the wholeness behind and identify primarily with the masculine or feminine gender. This is the awakening of sexuality. This is a second experience of Self with invincibility and vulnerability.

# Boy Age 15

## *Failing at School and Withdrawn*

This is a boy, between age fourteen and fifteen. He is from a family with five children. His father is very successful, but the children had suffered, as he had no time for them. This boy was failing at school and began to withdraw.

Never ask the child to do anything special. Ask them what they would like to do. Have many things available. Show them all of these things they could do. Never say, *"Maybe today we could do a drawing"*, etc. Everywhere else in their lives they are told what to do. This takes away their capacity to decide. Some have to learn to say what they would like to do. They must learn to *feel* what they would like to do.

It is completely wrong to say, *"Make a sandplay."* This way we touch their true needs. We can wait and be silent; we can talk. You have to have the patience to wait. Schizophrenics have a hard time feeling accepted. With one patient I just waited, then gave her a cup of tea. Provide the space where inner energies can come alive and express themselves.

You must have ultimate trust in the living being. If we do not we interfere with the process. You must be ready to receive what wants to be expressed. This is something that has to be expressed to relieve the situation. So we ask the client, *"What kind of impression does this make on you?"*

**Tray 1**
**Boy Age 15**

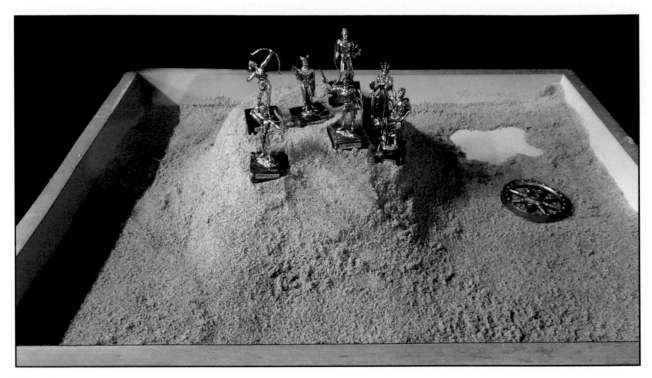

**Tray 1a**
**Boy Age 15**

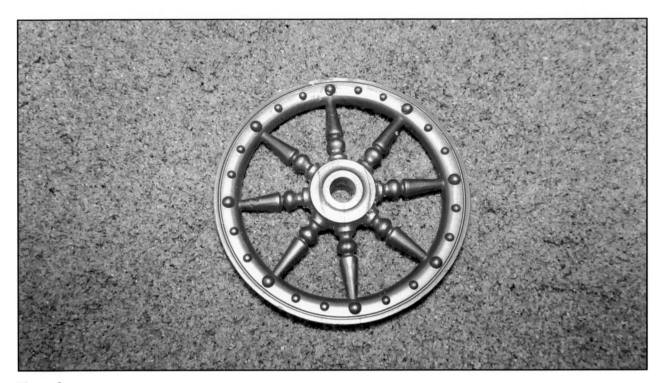

**Tray 1b**
**Boy Age 15**

Mount Olympus is in the center and he said the wheel is *"Sparta."*

What is your initial impression? *Isolated, barren, sad.*

Sparta is below the gods. There was a war in Sparta because Helen was raped. Helen is the feminine quality that is threatened. If one aspect of the Self is threatened, this gives us an image of an inner situation that is not complete. The difference in height between the mountain and Sparta speaks to his inability to extrovert.

The gods on Mount Olympus are far away from civilization. They are high up and are ruled by themselves. There is no connection between the lower and the higher. He said, *"The gods are reigning up there,"* so he is down in Sparta.

This boy is missing the guidance of his absent father. It is very important in puberty that the male child be able to follow the guidance of the father. The younger child follows the mother, because she is more tied to the home. The adolescent goes out of the home and follows the father. An adolescent that is not ready to go out is troubled.

This child is very introverted. The tendency of the child is to become like the father. Here this is very threatening to the boy. This is dangerous for him. His feminine side is being raped.

Sparta is seen to have a great value, because it is seen in a circular form. This shows that he would be able to make a connection between the feminine and the masculine to develop more fully.

He said that, *"The gods live up there and they also make mistakes."* This is working in the boy. He would also like to be up on Olympus, to achieve something like the image he has of his father. To do this, he would have to bring the two sides together.

The water is an opening to the unconscious – to the unconscious contents. The water is the container of many contents: fish, plants and other animals. There is much there that we do not see. Only when we dive into it do we see what is there. When the first picture shows the water, we may conclude that unconscious contents may arise sooner or later.

Many people say that the upper right is this and the lower right is that. This may be completely wrong. These are three dimensional images. This does not allow us to say left or right.

We do know from this picture that one part is completely empty. This means that there a lot that is hidden. This boy is thought to be very intelligent, but he could not bring it out to be seen. The introversion is the difficulty between the inner and the outer world. There is much more to be discovered.

There are seven gods on Olympus, and there are seven members in the family. Why did he use gods and not family members? It is coming from the unconscious. He is introverted. He is more expressive through the unconscious. When you are able to provide the *temenos* (sacred place set apart from ordinary time and space) the child enters deeper realms. His unconscious is aware of the problem. This is where the images come from. In any family problem, there is a problem beyond the conscious mind. We therefore need to give the unconscious contents the chance to show.

Puberty is the time between childhood and adulthood. They are in an empty space. They do not belong to either world. They are actually lost. This is a big gap.

**Tray 2**
**Boy Age 15**

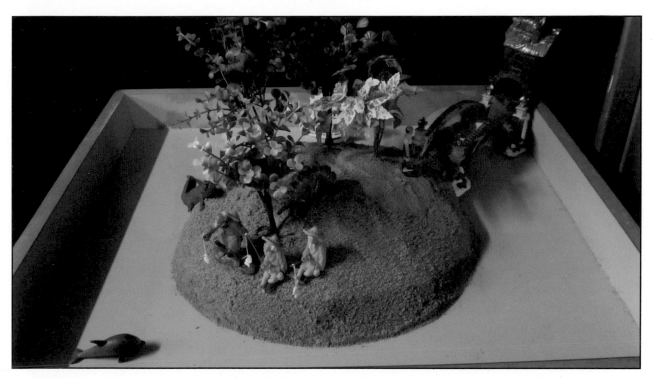

**Tray 2a**
**Boy Age 15**

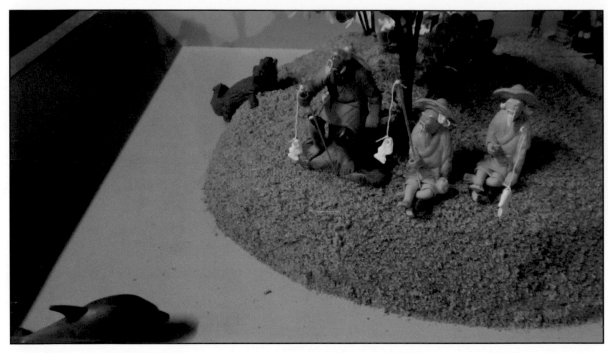

**Tray 2b**
**Boy Age 15**

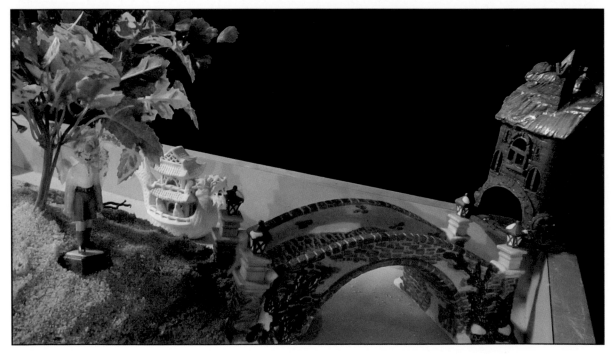

**Tray 2c**
**Boy Age 15**

The first impression is that we are at a deeper level of the unconscious. There is green here, but there is a threat. The alligator is the instinctive level and there is a threat from it. The dinosaur is a primeval, instinctual and archetypal threat. This has to do with puberty, because this is an archetypal situation. This is a threat to all mankind. It is the threat of becoming an adult. It could be a sexual threat. Dark elements are emerging and are aggressive. They are a threat from behind. He said he had a dream where he was walking home at midnight. To the left and the right of the path there were many snakes. This is the awakening of the sexuality.

The snake made Eve conscious of her femininity. The snake creeps on the floor. It cannot stand up. It can raise itself only a bit. This indicates that something is touched at the bottom of the body, in the tummy. Snakes are about transformation, because the skin changes. In some mythology the white snake is seen as a protector. Green brings something new. We always have to see which aspect is displayed at this moment for that particular person. Decide which is the most important aspect at the time.

The alligator can be a devouring mother. The client later said that his mother was overpowering him with love. In puberty there is a separation from the original protection of the mother. When the mother continues to protect the child as if he were still young, he feels threatened. This makes it difficult for him to move away from that protection. Sexuality is emerging at the same time. Mother is a woman. This can be a conflict. Here the alligator mother is warning him. He should become a man. He should pay attention to this situation.

They are fishing for a dolphin. This is an intelligent mammal. It is a beautiful content out of the unconscious which could belong to him. There is a great threat here that he cannot catch this fish.

Here we have the boat with the seven Chinese wise men. This boat is in the back. Remember that there were seven gods on Mount Olympus in Tray 1.

**The Seven Chinese Wise Men:**

1. The god of fishermen. He helps catch the fish.
2. The god of prosperity. He holds a bowl of rice.
3. The god of war has a spear in his left hand and a pagoda in his right.
4. A smiling old man carrying treasures. The rat comes near, but he has a magic hammer.
5. The goddess of music. This is a female deity. She sits on a dragon and has a lute with four strings.

6.  The god of long life has a crane and a turtle. The crane is longevity and the turtle is also about longevity.

7.  The god of contentment with a rat. The rat is about easy birth and many children.

There is a house here. Is this the house that he comes from, or the house that he is going to build? The seven gods may be bringing treasures to the new house.

The house on the edge can be something that is to come, or something that has been. The house and the bridge come up where the water was in Tray 1. Sometimes we cannot see what it is, but we can see several possibilities. Symbolic language has many possibilities. Just see what happens in the next tray.

We have seen that there may be a problem with authority – maybe with the divine qualities, also. He is actually fishing for that. The fish was Christ to the early Romans. "Fish," is *ICTUS* in Greek, Jesus Christos, the son of God the savior. He may be fishing for Christ.

## Tray 3
## Boy Age 15

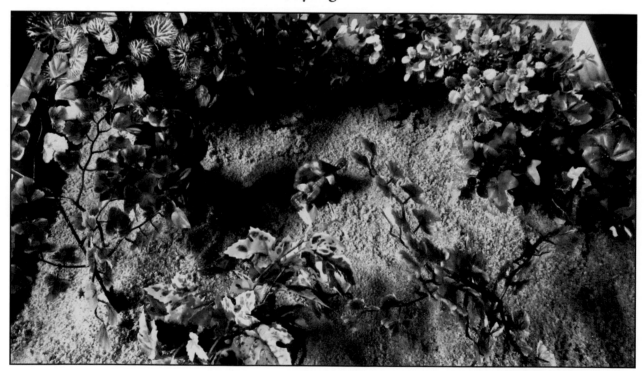

**Tray 3a**
**Boy Age 15**

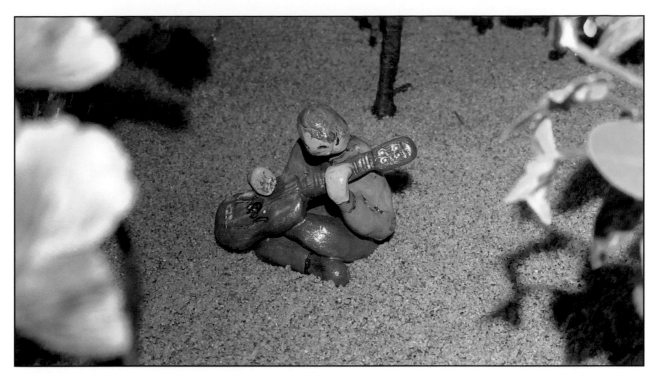

**Tray 3b**
**Boy Age 15**

Trees are in nature. This is a natural level of ourselves which we call the animal-vegetative. This is where instinctual life takes place. He has reached a place where there is no problem. He is there with his music at the animal level. This is an expression of the heart, of joy and well being. This is in contrast with other levels where he has to perform intellectually.

He is also very lonely. He is alone. This has to do with the kidney, the gall bladder, the deeper organs in ourselves.

In reaching this level, he has penetrated through the difficulty. This is like the state in the Garden of Eden, before they became aware, or conscious. In the Garden of Eden there is a snake that wants to bring consciousness. Here he is just by himself.

We also come nearer to the Self at these deeper levels. If he took this to consciousness, he would be very lonely. Experiencing it on a deeper level, he can enjoy it.

The young man is playing the guitar. This is a possibility for him to be artistic. This is a potential. If we have these possibilities within ourselves and do not use them, they can become very negative and disturbing. The energies that are not used can begin to rebel and disturb us.

First people become withdrawn, and then they draw within.

The woods are a level of the unconscious. There is darkness. One can discover many things here that we do not know. There are hidden possibilities. We can also say that there may be natural growth in this boy, because of the trees. The truth is without shadow. Because he was coming near to the essence, he is not yet able to communicate this. We can see the fertility that he lives with. This is really the sign of an introverted nature. An extrovert would likely not make this tray. But when an extrovert is able to penetrate to this layer, they may get in touch with this. He is coming into tune with his inner nature.

When you are working with the client, observe them making the pictures and feel what is going on.

Jung said that there is a synchronistic moment when what is happening in the outer world occurs at the same time in the inner world. If this takes place, then the psyche usually takes the next step in development. Because the therapist has the outer experience and can understand the client's inner experience simultaneously, this creates the synchronistic moment and the transformation takes place. If I am not able to see what they show me, there is the necessity for the client to play out the same situation many times until I get it. When I see the same energies playing out in the room, I have to ask what it is that I am not seeing.

**Tray 4**
**Boy Age 15**

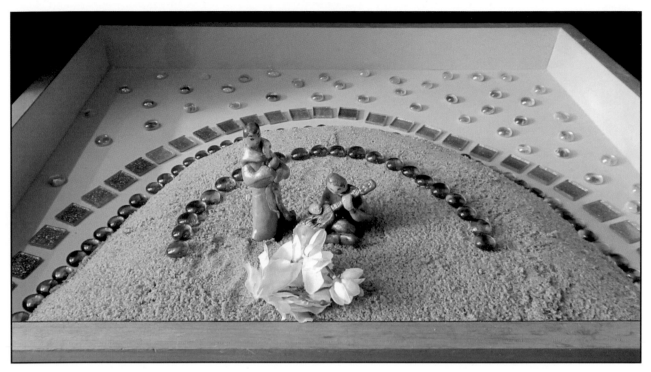

**Tray 4a**
**Boy Age 15**

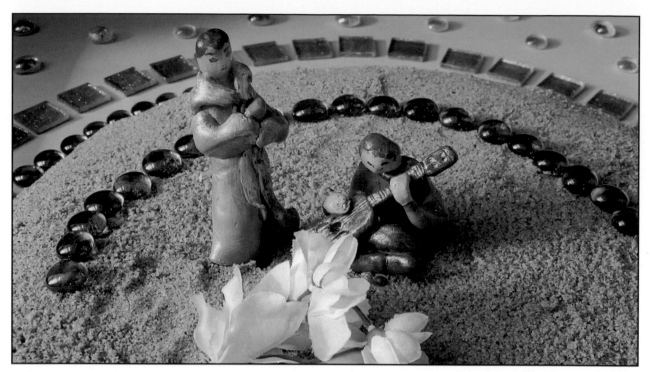

**Tray 4b**
**Boy Age 15**

This is the constellation of the Self. The masculine and the feminine are now in the world at the center of the cosmos. This is the union of the opposites. They stand in the center. Often heaven is shown in a circular form. This is being at one with the universe. He felt this, the essence of being one with the whole universe.

It is a half circle, because it is like standing on the earth and seeing the round firmament above and around him.

When I work with these children, there is always a crucial question about the divine quality. They stand in this space between child and adulthood. It is an empty space. In this empty space they look for something that gives them some sense of inner security. This can be gained by making contact with God. When they ask about God, ask, *"Where did you feel the best in your life? Did you ever have a really beautiful experience?"*

They all tell of an experience of getting in contact with the divine, with something that is greater than we are. When we make this contact, then the security begins to grow in the personality.

This is the essential question of puberty. When they contact this element, everything falls into place. Of course, they have to work with it and grow through different stages. From this point we grow and develop the personality.

This is also a preparation for the second half of life. Jung said his psychology is mainly experienced in the second half of life, after people have developed and achieved a goal. The question of the meaning of life usually comes after what has been lived through in the first half of life. Children who have undergone this experience in puberty will likely find their meaning in later life.

Puberty is the most important time in our lives. We need to give these children more time to find the meaning of their lives. When they contact the Self, they have a different attitude toward life. With drugs they think they get a glimpse of this. This does not last. What is lacking in our time is getting in touch with the essence. At the constellation of the Self many people burst into tears. They do not know that we are looking for such a thing until they find it.

This tray is the coming together of heaven and earth, of the masculine and the feminine. This union is experienced at this moment.

**Tray 5**
**Boy Age 15**

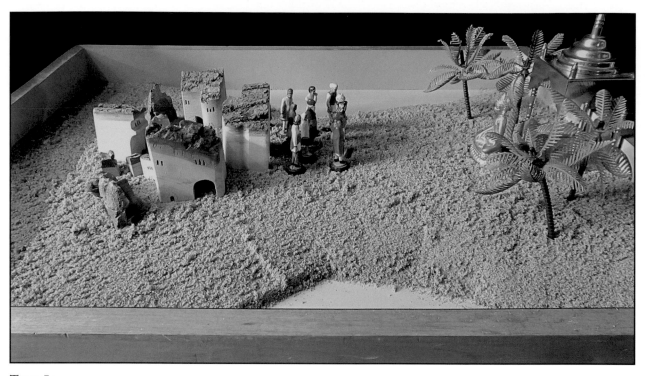

**Tray 5a**
**Boy Age 15**

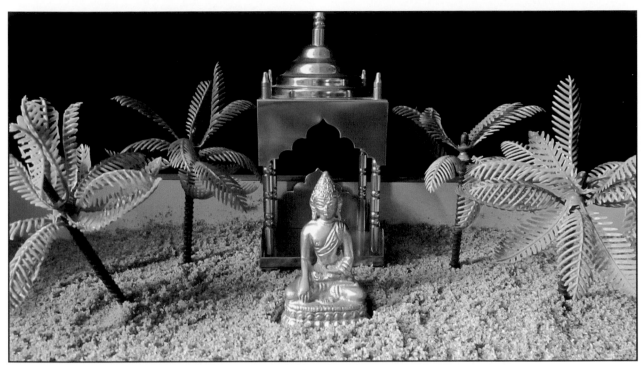

**Tray 5b**
**Boy Age 15**

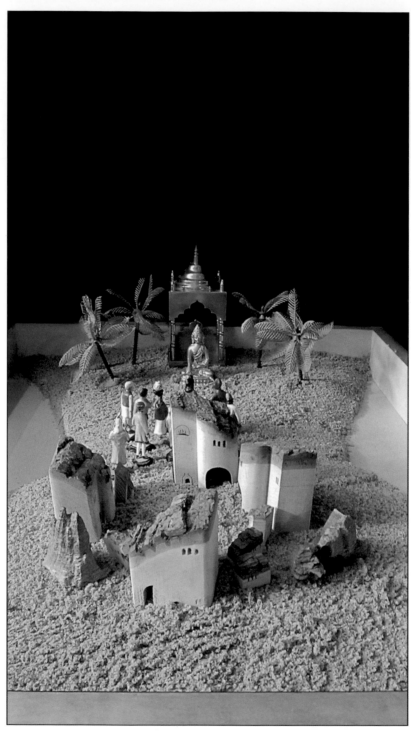

**Tray 5c**
**Boy Age 15**

Here he is on the way. The shape of the sand looks like a tree, looking right to left. It looks like a body, looking left to right.

I do not see water as the emotions, but as the unconscious. All parts of the Self are rallying around the divinity. The union of the opposites provides the totality. This moves people to feel that everyone should have this experience and be on the move.

Why does he have the Buddha here? The Buddha is the son of a king and queen and he is very spoiled. He never saw anything negative. Once his servant showed him the end of the palace grounds and he looked out into the world. He saw a very sick man, who was suffering with pain. He was very sorry to see this suffering, and became determined to find a way to relieve people of their suffering. He left the palace. He gave his crown and horse to his servant and instructed him to return to the palace. He meditated. After seven years of sitting under the bodhi tree, he was enlightened. He became clear about what the human being is and could be. All unconscious contents became clear to him. He was all-knowing and understood. He felt everyone should have the chance to become enlightened.

What we do with our work in sandplay leads a tiny little bit toward this clarity. The Buddha shows the path to God.

---

### *Participant Comment*

*Much inside is waiting to become conscious. Everyone should undergo such a process. He does not say this, but you can see that he sends everyone toward the Buddha.*

---

If the picture is a tree, the city is in the crown and the Buddha waits at the roots. This process brings us to our roots by penetrating to the depths of the unconscious.

Many youngsters have had the tendency to look to the Far East, because they could not find their answers here. When Westerners reach the depths of their unconscious, they use figures that are from a culture that is very far away. When Easterners penetrate into the depths, they very often use Christian symbols. People use figures from a different culture and geographically far removed. Greek figures can come when they are half way - half way between the East and the West. Everyone is born with the Buddha nature. We all have the capacity to become enlightened. The Buddha nature can be compared with the Self.

With our children, we only teach the intellectual side. We need to discover love, compassion and emotion. We do not evaluate children at school about this. This is why so many fail. It is often easier to accept something that comes from far away, rather than something that has been very near.

## Tray 6
## Boy Age 15

*The king will be buried here.*

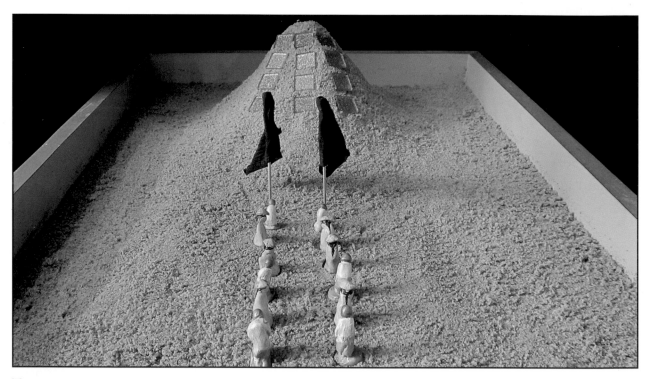

**Tray 6a**
**Boy Age 15**

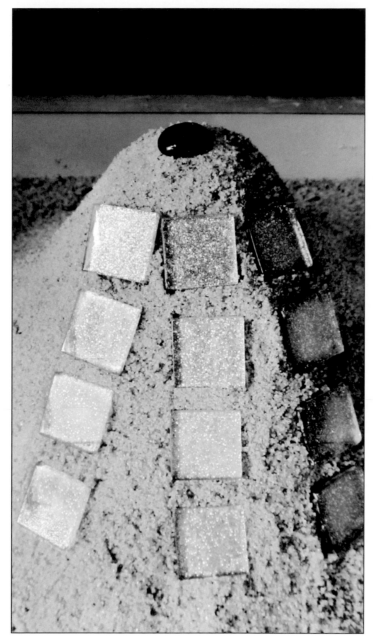

**Tray 6b**
**Boy Age 15**

*This is the Funeral for a King.*

The image of his father was too overpowering. It left him unable to be powerful himself. He has shown us that he must have an artistic quality. The father did not honor that. His father led a completely different life. He has to bury the image of the father. This is the archetypal father. He calls this *The Funeral for a King*. This is the pure masculine without the feminine quality. This must be buried now.

Then he is free to develop a different side of himself. He is still at the beginning of his ego development, because the ego emerges out of the Self. Here he must first bury an ego that is the figure of the overpowering king.

**Neumann spoke of four stages of ego development:**

1. The Constellation of the Self
2. The Animal-Vegetative Stage
3. The Battle Stage – Fighting. The ego must become strong and defend itself to be in competition in the outer world
4. Adaptation to the Collective

The red at the top of the burial mound may be the emergence of something new. Red would be feeling, emotion. This may be an indication of what has to come – the feeling function. The green is nature and the sensate function. Blue is the thinking function and yellow is the intuitive function.

---

## *Participant Question*

*Is the number of tiles he used significant symbolically?*

> I am not certain if we should interpret this tray this way. Sometimes figures are chosen because you have the number of figures that they need. Be careful with interpretations. If it is done properly, working with the sand helps prevent us from getting inflated. The image just appears; follow the process as it presents itself.

---

**Tray 7**
**Boy Age 15**

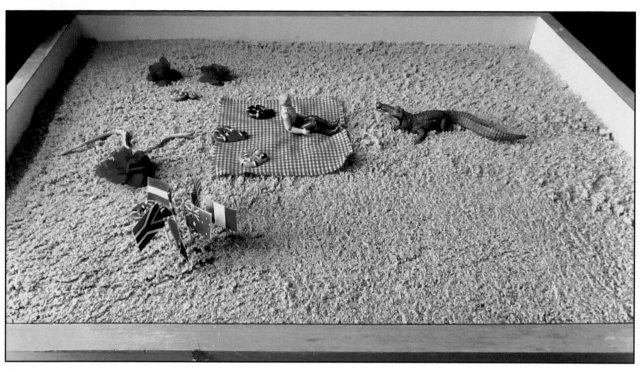

**Tray 7a**
**Boy Age 15**

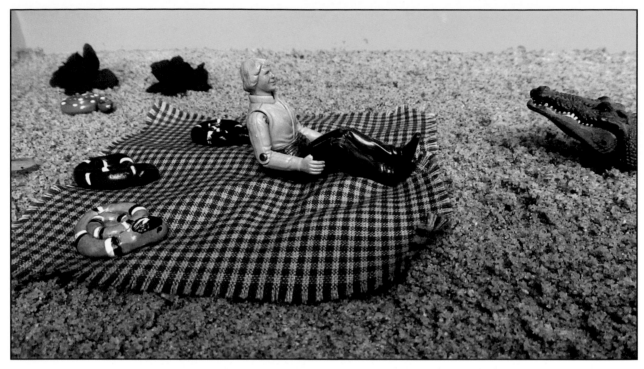

**Tray 7b**
**Boy Age 15**

There are several snakes here. The sexual development is touched. The natural instincts are facing the image of the devouring mother.

After the constellation of the Self, we touch the deep vegetative level in the Self. This is where the development really begins.

These are coiled snakes. This is the rising *kundalini*. (From yogic tradition, the latent feminine life force said to be coiled at the base of the spine) It is coiled two and one half times around itself. The awakening of the *kundalini* is the awakening of the feminine creative spirit. The crocodile is a devouring, threatening aspect. She could withhold this feminine quality that wants to develop in this young man. This is a big threat to him.

The manifestation of the Self gives us great courage. Very often after the manifestation of the Self it is possible to show the solution to the very difficult problem. This is the point of experiencing our totality and having the security to open to different possible solutions. Now he is able to show what his problem really is – the development of the masculine in a sexual form. At the same time the development of the feminine side, which may be the creative part of his later life is also indicated. The *kundalini*, the snake, has to be developed.

The red and white cloth is the spirit and the heart blending together. The red is an indication of love and emotion. Here is a confrontation of two kinds of feminine energy: the beginning of the creative one, and the devouring one. This is a psycho-physical image.

In Tibetan Buddhism the white and red is the creation of life. It is said that the beginning of all life comes out of a white and a red cell. These meet here. Here he is at the beginning of a new way of life.

Jung said that there is a personal unconscious which we reduce to at the beginning of our own lives, and there is a collective unconscious that is similar to all of mankind. We must learn about what things mean in other cultures. This is a picnic, nourishment. It is strife between two qualities of the feminine. The feminine quality that one experiences at this age can develop a spiritual side. The spirit is often seen as masculine, but the feminine *kundalini* spirit that rises from the base of the body to the head becomes spiritual. If this had been a girl the *kundalini* would also be feminine.

The upheavals and explosions in the world, the drugs, have to do with a feminine that has been neglected. With sandplay I have had the idea to develop the feminine in the human being again.

After the war, I lived in the Alps in a hut with my two sons and a nurse. That was all that was left for me. I began to think about what I wanted to do. The Jungs spent their holidays there. They decided that I should be an analyst, since I did not know what to do with myself.

We had found some baby foxes in a cave high up the mountain. One strayed out of the cave in the rain and caught a cold. Jung said I should study the fox. When I went to England I looked it up. The fox is shrewd, intelligent and always right, even when wrong. It is tricky with the bear and tricky with the hare. The fox murders the hare. The hare, the rabbit, was a friend of the fox in early Christianity.

The fox was also the doctor at the court of the lion. He always brought the hare, who was his friend. They worked together to cure the lion. Beginning with the twelfth century, the stories are different. Now the fox is fed up with the hare. He wants to be the only king and wants to murder the hare. He murdered the hare at the beginning of the thirteenth century.

So the fox is the intelligent, rational side and the hare is the feminine nature which is able to transcend during life. St. Francis took all of the sick animals under his care. He wanted to guide them toward heaven when they died. A healthy rabbit said he wanted to go with him to heaven. St. Francis said that was his choice and he could go. Then all of the animals died and found their paradise in heaven. But the rabbit was still alive and could not find paradise and said there must be no place for him there yet. St. Francis said he would ask God what to do with him. God told him to let the rabbit go down to earth, because he loves the earth like God does. So this is the story of the transcendence during life, which is symbolized during life. He loves the earth, but is able to transcend.

However, the hare is murdered at the beginning of the thirteenth century when Western philosophy began to orient toward the rational. This is where we are now. We have reached the end of this development. We lack the feminine, which is able to make the transition from earth to heaven. This is evident in this case.

Goethe took this story and made a poem of it. He describes the death of the rabbit. He knew where we were going in the Western culture. I took this as a warning that we must revive the feminine in the sense of the ability to become spiritual. I promised myself that I would try to develop the feminine in whoever came into my practice. This is the urgent need of our day.

---

## Goethe's Reineke Fox

*The king gives Reineke, the fox* (also called Renard) *his permission to seek absolution from the Pope in Rome for his misdeeds.*

"....Good and expedient is. I give thee gracious permission
Early to-morrow to start – the pilgrimage will I not hinder,
For, as it seems to me, from evil to good you are turning.
God the intention bless, and allow you to finish the journey!"

..."Leave is granted," the king replied; and then he commanded
All the lords of his Court to go for a part of the journey
With the pretended pilgrim, as escort. In pain and in sorrow
Meanwhile Brown (*Bruin, the Bear*) and Isegrim (*the wolf*) both were lying in prison.

Thus had Reineke once again the love of the monarch
Fully regained, and went from the Court in the fulness of honour,
Seemingly bound with wallet and staff to the Sepulchre Holy,
Where he had just as little concern as a maypole in Aachen.
Different quite were his designs

...his malice he could not forego, but said in departing:
"Gracious sir, take very good care that the couple of traitors
Do not escape you, but keep them well tied up in the prison.
Were they free, with scandalous deeds they'll not be contented.
Danger threatens your life. Sir king, fail not to be careful."

So he went on his road with quiet and pious demeanour,
With an innocent look, as if he knew not another.
Then arose the king and back he went to the palace,
All the animals following thitherwards. As he had ordered,
They had accompanied Reineke part of the way on his journey,
And the rogue had maintained an anxious and mournful demeanour,
So that many a kind-hearted man was moved to compassion.
Lampe, the hare, in especial was very much grieved, as the rascal
Cried, "Dear Lampe, we must, o! must we indeed be divided?
Might not you and Bellyn, the ram, to-day have the kindness
On my road to come a little bit further? Upon me
By your company you will confer a very great favour.
Honest, good folk you are withal, and pleasant companions.
Ev'ry one speaks of you well, and this would redound to my honour.
You are religious and saintly in morals, and both live correctly,
Even as I in the convent lived. Contented with green herbs,
Hunger you always appease on leaves and on grass, never asking
Either for bread or meat, or other particular viands."
Thus the weakness of both with praise he managed to flatter.
Both went on with him till they came to his dwelling, and looked on
Malepartus, the fortress; and Reineke said to the ram there:
"Bellyn, remain outside, and enjoy the grass and the herbage
To your heart's content. Upon these hills are afforded
Many plants that are good for the health and of excellent flavour.
Lampe with me I take, but beg him to give consolation
To my wife, who already is troubled, and when she discovers
That I must go as a pilgrim to Rome, will be almost despairing."
Sweet were the words of the fox to the pair, wherewith to deceive them.
Lampe he led inside, where he found the sorrowing vixen,
Lying beside her children, with great anxiety cumber'd,

For she did not believe from the Court that Reineke ever
Home would return. Now when she saw him with staff and with wallet,
Strange did the matter appear, and she said to him: "Reynard, my darling,
Tell me, then, how it has gone with you, and all that befell you?"
And he said: "I was judged already and bound as a captive,
But the king his mercy bestowed, and gave me my freedom.
And as a pilgrim I came away, and as hostages left there
Brown and Isegrim both. Meanwhile the king has presented
Lampe in compensation, to do with him as it may please us.
For the king declared at last with excellent judgment:
'Lampe it was that acted the traitor.' Thus certainly he has
Signal correction deserved, and must make me an ample atonement."
Lampe with terror transfix'd these threatening words apprehended,
And in bewilderment hastened to save himself by escaping.
Reineke quickly block'd up the doorway; the murderer seized him,
Wretched thing, by the throat, who loud and shrill for assistance
Screamed: "O Bellyn, help me! oh! help! I am done for; the pilgrim
Murders me.' Yet no long did he cry, for Reineke soon had
Bitten him through the throat. It was thus his guest that he welcomed.
"Come now," he said, "let us eat him quickly; the hare is a fat one,
Good in flavour, too. In soothe, he is now for the first time
Somewhat of use, silly fool! I swore long ago I would do it.

Canto VI
*Reineke Fox, West-Eastern divan, and Achilleid*
Johann Wolfgang von Goethe (1749-1832)
Original Publisher: London, G. Bell and sons, 1890

---

In the Far East, the rabbit and the fox remained good friends. In China they say that when the hare dies, the fox cries. In Tibet, the fox and the hare have the same qualities. Tibet is right between the East and the West and has both qualities. We must learn more about their philosophy.

The feminine is not the emotional, concentrated energy. It is compassion, true love, which can develop to a true spirit. It is the evolution of true love to spirit. In *The Little Prince*, the fox showed the prince the rose and he learned about love.

The flags are used at times of celebration. They are a symbol of a collective identity. This is a celebration of a new beginning. There is a lot of tension which he can endure now. He can develop his own manhood, because he can deal with the devouring mother. This is a very important part of puberty – the transition from the innocent boy to a man. If this does not happen at this time, there are difficulties with men.

At the same time, it is just as important to feel that the feminine aspect must grow for him to become whole. At the moment of the manifestation of the Self, all of the forces are kept in a nucleus. Then all of the development begins to open and flower - both masculine and feminine. That is why we see the feminine here in the form of a snake. It may still have a poisonous look. We must be aware of this psycho-physical development of the youth to understand what is going on. If we do not, something which wants to bloom has to hold back and it becomes rebellious.

We think of the feminine as Kwan Yin or Mary. To understand what the feminine of today has lost, we have to look back to what the feminine meant in early Christianity. Today, with feminism women want to be like men. The first feminine picture in the man is the mother. If she is not a real mother, the man cannot develop a pure feminine side. We must be fully feminine to be appreciated by a man. It is very important to know what the woman's task is. There would be less tension in the world if the feminine were more valued.

There is a Tibetan Buddhist meditation to unite the masculine and the feminine. A glowing thread starts from the lowest part of the body (chanting) *Ahhhhhhhh*. This grows hotter as you meditate. It moves up to the head and meets the (chanting) *Hummm*. It melts the hum, merges them together and they move down to the heart. This is a wonderful image of the value of both the masculine and the feminine. If the heart is in the center of the spirit, it is the center for love. This is how we can really understand each other - through this place.

## *Participant Question*

*When we work with a sand tray and do not know what it is about, what is lost when we do not have an interpretation?*

It is dangerous to have an immediate interpretation. We have to experience it with the client. We must reflect on it later. The important thing is to experience it with the person. It is the sharing of the experience that is the most important.

## Tray 8
## Boy Age 15

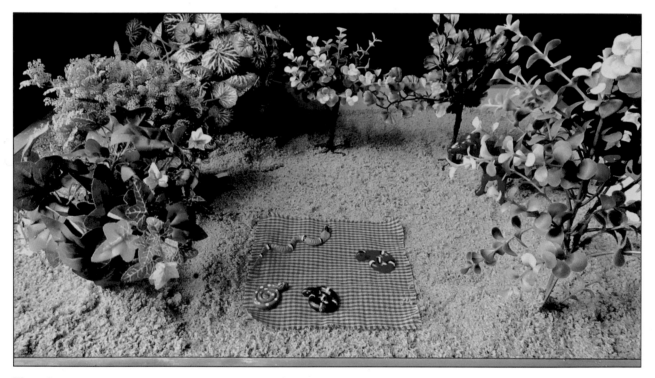

**Tray 8a**
**Boy Age 15**

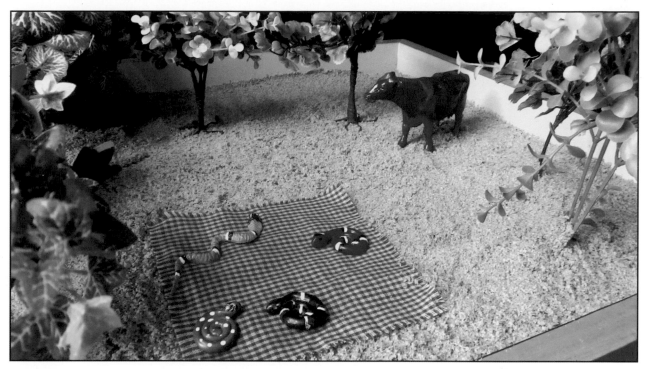

**Tray 8b**
**Boy Age 15**

Here we have a red cow. The crocodile has turned into the cow. The fire is incorporated into the nurturing feminine.

His trays have alternated between being barren and having trees. The barren trays show a new beginning which has not been nurtured. Then the tray with the trees shows that the nature within him is working to develop.

There is much more concentration here. The feminine is not diffused throughout the tray as it was in the last one. The feminine is coming together in an orderly way. This is why we should not interfere by giving interpretation. I trust that the healing side of the psyche takes over the healing process when I give it the space. This side knows more than we can intellectually know.

You see, by itself the crocodile turns into a nurturing element.

We have four snakes. There are the four elements in the body. According to Jung there are four functions – thinking, feeling, intuition and sensation. The body is made of four elements – earth, water, fire and air. The fifth is the spiritual side that nourishes all. It is important that order be brought into the elements.

The new element of the cow enters. The cow is at a distance. It is new and is coming in to the center. She is in the same position where the crocodile stood before.

There was a lot of talking between his trays. He did not do them weekly after the manifestation of the Self. Usually when the manifestation of the Self has taken place, there can be more talking.

Always see the parents first. You want to know why they are bringing the client in. What do they expect? And what is wrong? You want to understand their complaints. Then I tell them that I will see the child, but I want to protect the free and protected space. So there should be no interference from outside from the parents or the teachers. If they agree to this, I take the child. I also tell them that there could be situations where the child seems to get worse. I tell them that they can call me. But if it becomes necessary to see the parents, I ask the child if they will allow it.

So sometimes I ask the child if I can show some pictures to the parents. Then I explain them in a simple way to the parents. The unconscious of the child speaks to the unconscious of the parents. This is very powerful. This is how we treat the families. I think that if we work seriously with one part of the family, it usually has a good influence on the other family members. It is important to *not* involve the whole family in treatment. I feel that there is much hurt done with this. (Family therapy) We all have to work as we feel we must. Work your truth.

**Tray 9**
**Boy Age 15**

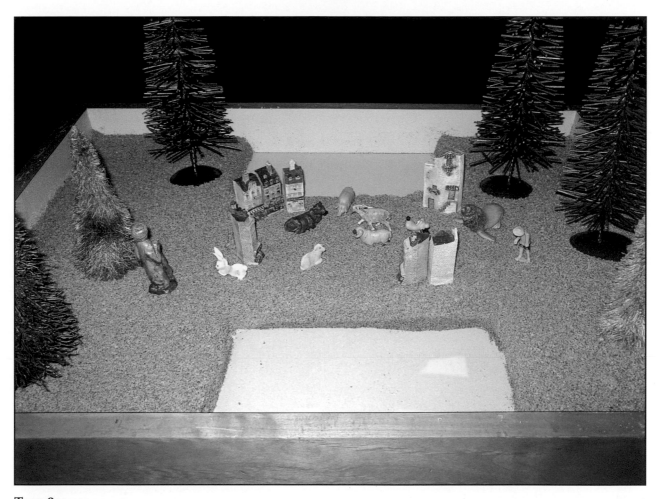

**Tray 9a**
**Boy Age 15**

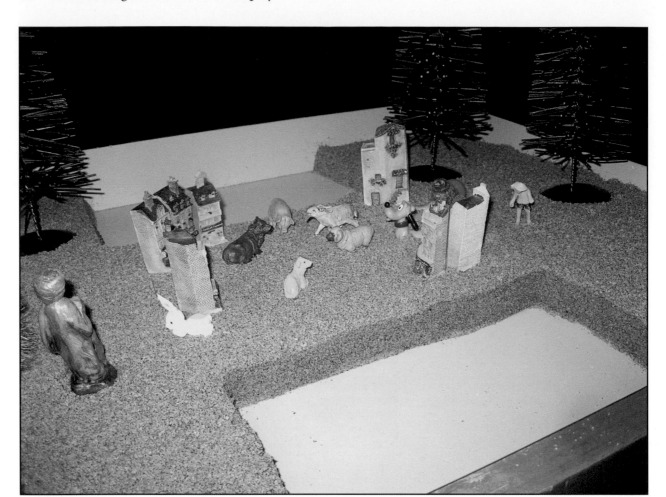

**Tray 9b**
**Boy Age 15**

The city is full of animals. These are more domesticated animals. He has moved from the woods to the city. This is the deeper side of the unconscious going toward more consciousness.

The sea lion is the animal that has come from the depths and now sits on the land. This indicates a transition between different levels of himself.

The lambs are new-born and vulnerable. They are associated with God.

There are white and black cats. Cats do what they need to do; they are purely instinctual.

The white rabbit is running toward the left. He begins to be more aware of the instinctual forces, which are concentrated in the middle. White is the tendency toward the spirit. The rabbit that is able to make contact with God during life. In The Chinese say that, in a former incarnation, Buddha was a white rabbit. The other animals did not like him. He asked them what he should do to make them happy. They told him they would make a huge fire and that he had to jump in to it. If he came out as white as when he went in, they would believe he was a special rabbit. He jumped in and came out just as white as he had been. The other animals had great respect and gave him a special place in the moon, where he constantly makes the elixir of life. See if the person who uses this symbol has an inclination for a spiritual direction.

When someone goes very deep, they use symbols from the opposite end of the world. When they do not go so far down, they use symbols from nearer by. The farmers indicate that he is becoming more and more conscious, because they are not so remote.

These pine trees have a phallic form, a masculine quality. The feminine tree has a round crown. The rabbit and the man are heading toward it.

The pig can dig for truffles, for the treasure. He brings the treasure out of the earth. Pigs have to do with fertility. In Greek mythology this is associated with Demeter, the earth goddess.

Pluto is the dog and rules the unconscious.

The bridge is between two realms. This may be a connection from the unconscious side to the more conscious side.

The tiles are made of earth, water, fire and air. This is devoid of the gods, now. It is a city that is brought down to earth. Sparta has come alive for this boy.

**Tray 10**
**Boy Age 15**

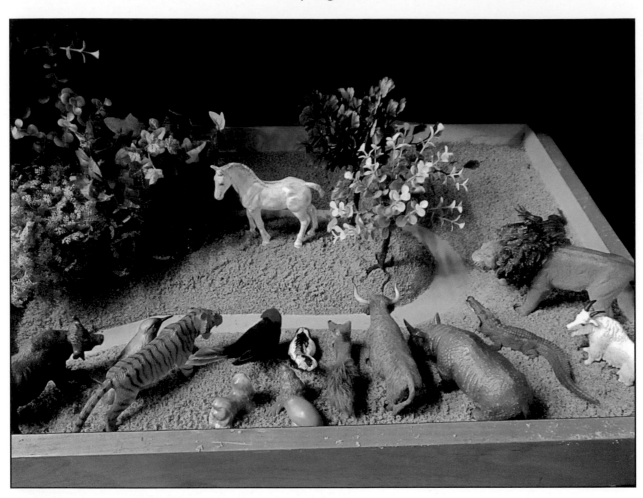

**Tray 10a**
**Boy Age 15**

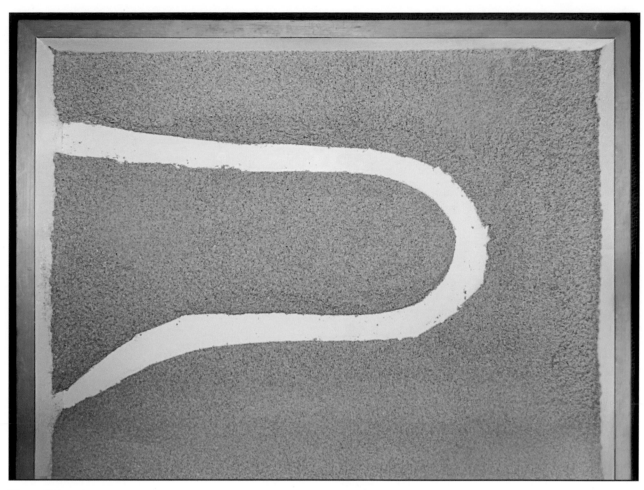

**Tray 10b**
**Boy Age 15**

*All of these animals come to get advice from the white horse.*

The white horse is in connection with the divine quality. This can be spirit, but it is more the divine quality. Mohammed rides on a white horse to heaven. Many divinities are connected with the white horse. There are temples in Japan where they keep white horses. Be careful not to simply say that it is a spiritual symbol. It is an animal with a divine quality.

Here his instincts begin to turn toward a spiritual side. The horse has tremendous energy.

There are many animals, both domestic and wild. All are his energies; there are many kinds that he begins to feel awakening. Some he can guide like the domestic animals, but some are wild. The wild energies that we see come up can be tamed by the white horse. He needs the divine quality to integrate these wild energies. All of these energies have been awakened in the manifestation of the Self. They get stirred up. They come to the divine quality for advice, to be tamed. In Zen, the wild ox has to be tamed. The ox is the mind.

The island is phallus shaped. The boy begins to feel the power and strength of his phallus. The phallus is masculine, the fluid, the water is feminine. This is a union of the masculine and feminine in the center with the horse. This is the coming together, a union. This is a numinous experience. This, again, is a symbol of the manifestation of his totality. This is the lingam in the yoni. This is a sacred image.

The lion and tiger are more powerful than the white horse, but they also come to ask advice of the white horse.

In Hinduism, *Kalki* is the tenth incarnation of Vishnu. He is supposed to arrive on a white horse. Perhaps the white horse is a symbol of something great, something divine to come.

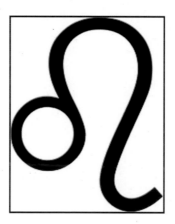

**Astrological Sign of Leo**

The astrological sign of Leo, the sun, is the same shape as the waterway. It is a symbol of becoming conscious. The individuation process has to do with becoming conscious of our possibilities. This is what this boy is doing.

---

## *Participant Question*

*Should we look to see ourselves in the client's trays?*

I do not like to see myself in the picture. If I see myself it would not be humble. Do not see yourself as the one that guides the process. You provide the space so the process can take place. Our help is to provide the empty, protected space where the process can happen. Do not interfere with the process by wanting something or directing something. We must have tremendous respect to observe this process taking place. To see a human being grow and develop their potentials is something very wonderful.

---

**Tray 11**
**Boy Age 15**

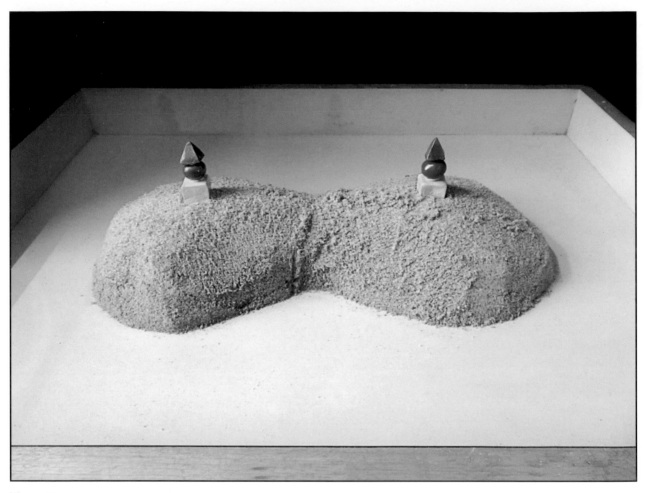

**Tray 11**
**Boy Age 15**

This is the coming together of the masculine and the feminine.

The triangle is fire. In Tibetan Buddhism, the square is earth, and the circle is water. These symbols are in tune with the body. Tibetan medicine says that when the elements are in tune with each other, the body is healthy.

The earth element concerns the regenerative organs. The color associated with it is yellow. Water is associated with the gall bladder and kidneys and is white. Fire concerns the heart functions of warmth and feeling and is red. Air is the breath and speech and is green. Ether is space and the color is blue.

| Element | Body Correlate | Color |
|---------|----------------|-------|
| Earth | Regenerative Organs | Yellow |
| Water | Gall Bladder Kidneys | White |
| Fire | Heart Function Warmth & Feeling | Red |
| Air | Speech & Breath | Green |
| Ether | Space | Blue |

Here he brings together the triangle, the circle and the square on a higher level, as they are on the breast. This is the nurturing feminine element in contrast with the devouring mother crocodile we saw earlier. This may be the mother, or his feminine quality. The feminine quality which was threatening at the beginning has now become nurturing.

Here we have two constructions - two in one. This is Tao, the sense of wholeness. According to Jung, the number two indicates that the person sooner or later becomes more conscious of what was lacking. Here he feels the growing feminine in himself. This was lacking at the beginning. The feminine has been thwarted since the thirteenth century. Since then the rational side has overwhelmed the feminine and the feminine has been neglected.

At this point he began to be very creative. He was painting and writing. He was nourishing his intellect with the feminine. Now he has his first experience with girls.

What is in the tray has not yet completely developed in the person. It shows what is going to happen in the person. If we see it in the tray, we can be certain that it will come. Many clients come back much later to see the slides that they made. Sometimes people say that all that has been made in the trays is realized over the years. The psyche shows the path in the trays. This is the path that is indicated by birth.

Here the shape of the sand resembles a fertilized cell dividing. Sand and water are two basic elements like the earth and water. This helps to nourish the feminine quality. The earth is feminine. If we talk and try to explain, we work with the air element and leave out the water.

Richard Wilhelm said, that Christ was born out of the spirit and became material, therefore the West has developed materially. On the other hand, Buddha was born of the family and meditated and developed spiritually. Therefore, the East has developed spiritually.

He felt that both sides have reached their limits and that now we have to come together. We must bring the spirit and the material together. The East has developed the material side with tremendous speed. The Japanese children are not wanting to go to school now. The East has been introverted and spiritualized for hundreds of years. When the Western ideas, rationality and technicalities came in, they had an empty mind to take it in. They took in all of what we know in just a few years. Now these children refuse to take in anymore. They cannot take in any more. It came in too fast.

---

## *Participant Questions*

*What are the dimensions of the sand tray?*

The tray should be 28.5x19.75x2.75 inches inside measurements.

*When are we ready to practice sandplay?*

Jung said to never stop working on yourself. This work has to do with a humble attitude in the face of what the human being can do. We are able to provide the empty space, in the sense of the fullness of the emptiness. Then we have the respect of the personality and for the person and for the totality of life.

I never expect anything. When we do not expect anything, we have to *be*. We have to live the moment completely. We must be present at each moment with all that we have.

*Should we have figures of different proportions?*

All of the figures should be all about the same size.

---

# Tray 12
## Boy Age 15

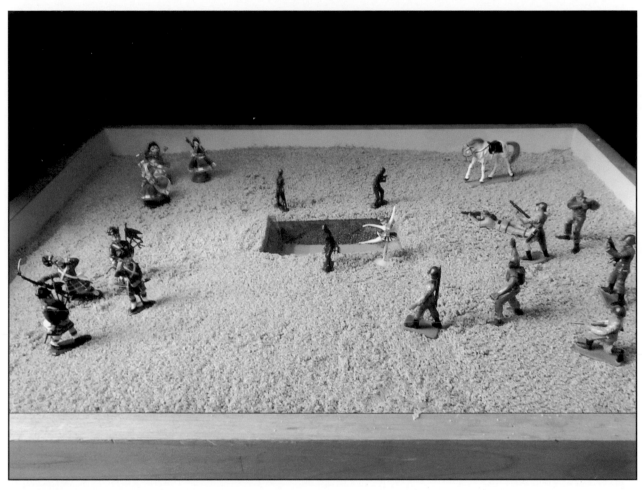

**Tray 12a**
**Boy Age 15**

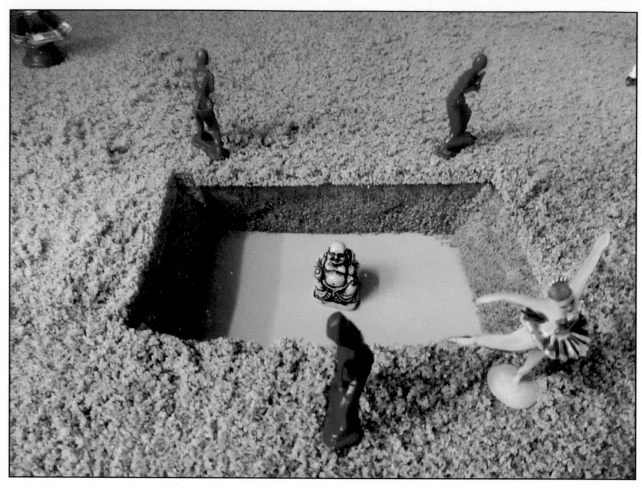

**Tray 12b**
**Boy Age 15**

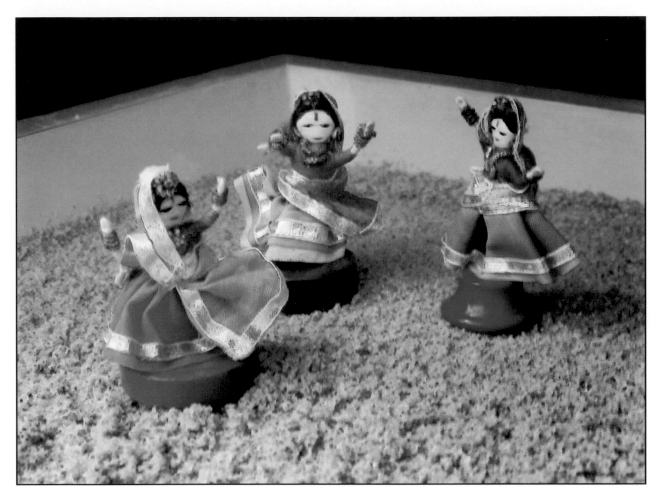

**Tray 12c**
**Boy Age 15**

*"This is the battle of all battles, which will have an influence on the world."*

Here there is a battle within the battle. The battle is on the surface, yet inside he has peace. This battle is with the outer world. A discussion with the world can be in fighting terms or in understanding terms. This is more of a discussion, a debate, than a fight. It is a fight to get accepted, or integrated into the world.

This is an inner fight. He feels secure within himself. The battle can go on. It is interesting that he says it will change the world. This fight is in participation with all of those around.

The arrangement of the three red soldiers is a downward pointing triangle. This is the feminine. The upward pointing triangle is the masculine, fire.

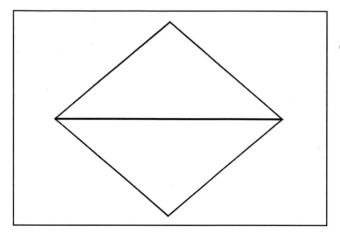

**Masculine as Upward Pointing Triangle**
**Feminine as Downward Pointing Triangle**

The center of the tray is the main concern here. With the Buddha underneath, he wants to say, *"I have this secure spot."*

After the manifestation of the Self, the Self appears again as an image in the following sequence of pictures. Jung said that when the Self is strong, it guides the process. There is always a relationship between the ego world and the Self inside.

It may be that they were aiming for the Buddha. Buddha went into the desert to meditate. Out in the wilderness, when he was near enlightenment, he was threatened by the darkness. We often see this as many aggressors coming toward the Buddha with spears. They just turn around, as they cannot hit him. He is too strong. The attitude of the client and what is coming out of his unconscious is what counts. I felt that this experience was so strong, that nothing could harm him.

The glass is made of sand, fire and water, and it is protective. The Buddha can be seen. This is an integration into the world. He was an outsider. Now he begins to fight for integration. The inner Self is untouched, unmoved by the play, the *maya* (delusion) of the world. He does not fear having this fight.

The horse here may not have any special meaning. Perhaps it is coming into the battle with power. There are many feminine elements mixed in with this battle. Life goes on within the battle. Here is a dancer. At the beginning we saw him playing the guitar. It may be that the dancer is showing that his artistic talents are becoming more evident. When he was about nineteen, he went abroad to attend a dancing school.

The center of the tray figures prominently, because he is looking for his center. The triangular shape may mean that he is near the center, but not there yet, whereas the square would be being at the center. Not always, however. He is struggling to find the center. It may have been touched already, but he is not always there. Here, the Buddha shows the center.

Do we need to know who is going to win the battle? No. This is not possible. With what he said about the picture, we can hope that he will achieve a better integration with the world, but we cannot say for certain. We have to be able to be open to take what is happening at the moment. If we think it should be like this or that, it will influence the client. We can have hope, but we must leave the open space. When one of us is changed, the whole world is changed.

---

## Maya

Maya is the name of the Hindu goddess who sustains the illusion of duality as reality. The word maya is translated as illusion, indicating that what we see and refer to as the manifest universe is actually just a projection of limited consciousness, behind which exists the permanence of ultimate, undivided Being.

---

## Tray 13
## Boy Age 15

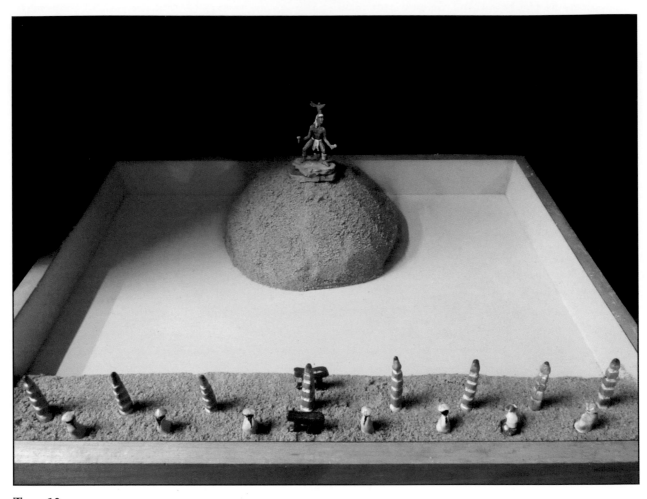

**Tray 13a**
**Boy Age 15**

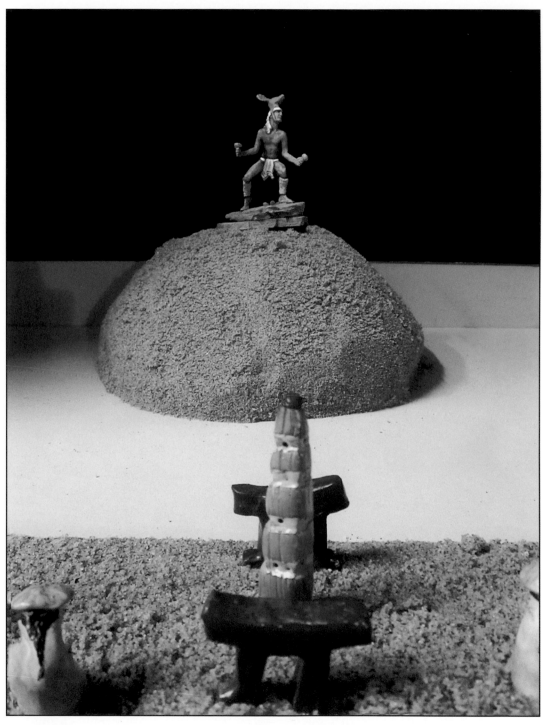

**Tray 13b**
**Boy Age 15**

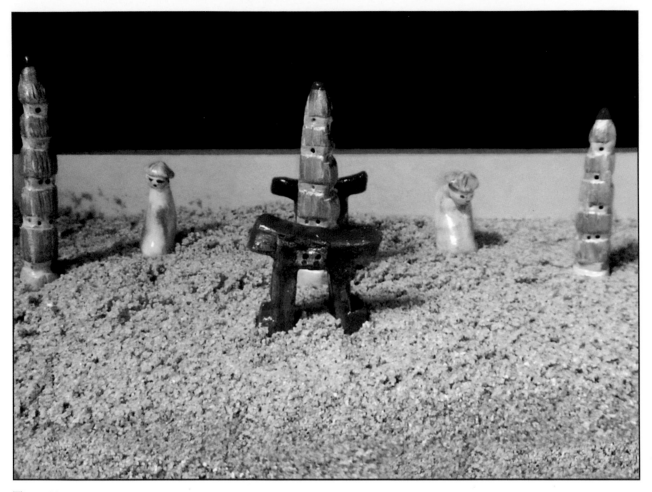

**Tray 13c**
**Boy Age 15**

*"They are all looking for the spirit of the mountain."*

This is like the tray where the animals came to the horse for advice. This is now a humanized figure. There is more order. These people work in the fields. They will know more about the spirit of the mountain than will the city people. There is the same up and down difference as in the first tray with Mount Olympus. Now there is some resolution, some cooperation.

Here is a five-story pagoda. Now he has achieved the five elements within himself and is approaching completion. In the East, they know that one can reach a spiritual attitude only through the body. The five-story pagoda shows the five elements in the body: earth, water, fire, air and spirit. These five elements are the symbol of the divine, because when you are able to reach the spirit through the body, then you are secure. This is the connection of the body and the spirit.

These are Chinese workmen. They know that they connect the body and the spirit. They work with the earth and look toward the spirit on the mountain. This is the relationship between earth and heaven. The client sensed this strongly and it gave him an inner security. He needed to express this.

When Buddha experienced enlightenment, there were no witnesses around, so he touched the earth to be his witness. The spirit is always connected with the earth.

We have a mountain and the water, the unconscious. When we reach the mountain, we cannot leave the depths. He is feeling comfortable with both the consciousness and the unconscious. He feels more complete.

All of the buildings are one quarter turned toward the mountain. This is an integration of fire with the feminine.

The medicine man is a healer. The healing comes from the mountain. Now he is at a higher level of consciousness and acts from this healing. The client feels a healing within himself.

The many pagodas show the strength and force within him. This may be the reason he chose several of the same symbol. This city is so much richer and stronger than the original Sparta. He did not accept the Greek gods on Olympus, saying that they made their mistakes just like people. Now there is a healer up there.

Puberty is a very powerful time. This work helps the client move through this time with power, rather than being frustrated by it. Puberty is an experience of the gap between childhood and the adult. It is like the *pingala* and the *ida*. (From the Hindu tradition – Two energy channels through which *prana*, or life force, moves)

There would be much less upheaval in adolescence if we would provide for more security within the child. This insecurity causes so much fear and tension. We cannot change the world for these young people, but perhaps we can give them a bit more strength to deal with it.

Often the clients try to come out and be who they are, but the parents try to keep this under wraps. In his early work, Jung felt that the client lived the unsolved problems of the parents, so he did not think it was a good idea to work with the child. He was right, but how many parents will come in? The work with the child will affect the parents, also.

---

## Participant Questions

*What do we do about adolescents who do not want to come in for therapy?*

A child of fifteen or sixteen has to make his or her own decisions to come into therapy, or not. We must let them choose themselves. We must tell the parents this. If the parents say that the child will not like to come in, then you can suggest that the parents work – not because there is anything wrong, but so they can understand the child better. This can be very effective.

The energies working in puberty are very strong and powerful. Adolescents are looking for something that is stronger than them. They need something they can rely on and trust. If the parents are insecure and the children cannot rely on them during this time, they do not have the strength and security that they must have. These types of parents have not resolved their anxieties and insecurities. We must reflect on the kind of atmosphere that we provide for the client.

*How do we direct adolescents to do a tray?*

There is always a danger in telling someone that they can "make a tray." This gives them the idea that something has to be displayed. Just introduce the sand. Say it has a good feeling and can be moved. Do this at the beginning, especially. We do not want them to think that they have to make a representation of something. They may have the idea that they have to make something from their daily life. It is just the opposite. You can ask how they feel when they touch the sand. You can say that sometimes hills and lakes appear. You can say that sometimes people put in a tree to show that it is nature. Be very careful.

*What does it mean when clients do not touch the sand?*

When people do not touch the sand and just put their figures in, it could be an underlying psychotic tendency. The fear of touching the earth, of getting in contact with deeper levels, is a fear of activating the unconscious. If people will not touch the sand, just let it be like this.

*Is it appropriate to use sandplay with psychotic patients?*

Sandplay can be a dangerous tool with psychotic tendencies. These can break out and be overwhelming. We must be very careful to recognize this.

*What do we do with an isolated client who always does trays of daily life?*

The client may be very isolated in his life and have no one with whom to share his daily activities. This is true, but the tray may also represent his inner life. Look at why the client chooses to talk about the particular symbols that they use. The symbols that they are choosing may tell you about something that is coming from within. If you begin to understand that, then perhaps a synchronistic moment will occur. Listening can be very creative.

Can we really listen and take in what is told, or do we listen and think about what we are going to say? Listen like a vessel that can always receive. Through this creative listening the inner motivation is activated. Leave the reasoning aside.

We cannot expect that everyone will play in the sand.

*Is it alright to put the tray up against the wall?*

Always keep the tray by itself. People should be able to move completely around the tray.

*What is the significance of repetitive trays?*

Repetitive trays indicate that I do not understand what it is that the child is trying to tell me. It is like a dream that keeps coming up until we get what the dream is trying to tell us.

*Is it alright to use sandplay with clients with a weak or needy ego structure?*

When the client undergoes the manifestation of the Self, the ego grows through the various stages. A needy ego is not in contact with the Self. These are people who cannot take much, because there is no support at the bottom of the whole personality. Today we find that most of us are not completely in contact with the Self. To strengthen is to make a connection with the Self. Then difficulties can be endured when they come up. This all depends on our inner structure.

*What can we do about being isolated as a therapist?*

To Jung I complained that I was all alone. Jung said that he has been alone his entire life, but that each child that comes to me brings me something.

When I finished my training, there were no analysts for children. Jung's work is for the second half of life. I said I could not work with children, asking them about dreams, visions, paintings, etc. I did not think I could do this, unless I found something that would allow me to recognize the unconscious in the child. There was a big congress of psychiatrists in Zurich. There I saw two sand trays. They belonged to Margaret Lowenfeld, who used them for diagnosis. I told her that I would like to come and study with her. She said I would have to stay three years. So, I had her talk with Mrs. Jung, who was my analyst at the time. After that talk, she said I could come any time I wanted.

What she did was fascinating - she just had them do a picture every now and then to check and see how the client was coming along. But she did not see the sequence that was developing. I was able to see many things that she did not. She was interested in this. When I went home, I began playing with the children with this. I made notes and photos of each tray and what the child said. At the beginning I saw that there was a development, but I could not yet trace what was going on.

Two years later I was asked to come to the United States to talk about this. I studied the pictures and saw that there was a similar theme of development with each child. This was how it started.

I felt that we really must observe the path that is shown in the sand pictures. I believe that the path is indicated by birth. It is about where we should go and could go. Through our one-sided development, we deviate from this path. We take a side path. In all of the cases, the problem unfolded until they came to the Self. They showed me what the dark side was, and then they entered the deeper levels of the Self. We find the path, which is in connection with the Self. The Self is guiding the process and the difficulties disappear. They may develop new problems, but they can handle them with this strengthening of the Self.

We see that people live out what they have shown in their trays over the course of time. Therefore there is an indication of a path. It is very important to find this path. Often when we are under stress, it is because we are trying to follow a path that is not really ours.

I was grateful that I was called to the US. In Europe, people do not respond to this. But here people are very curious.

*What are the differences between working with Easterners and Westerners?*

The Eastern and the Western minds are different, but the process is the same. Our outer lives are different, but we discover similar paths inside. We just use different symbols and expressions to show it.

---

**Tray 14**
**Boy Age 15**

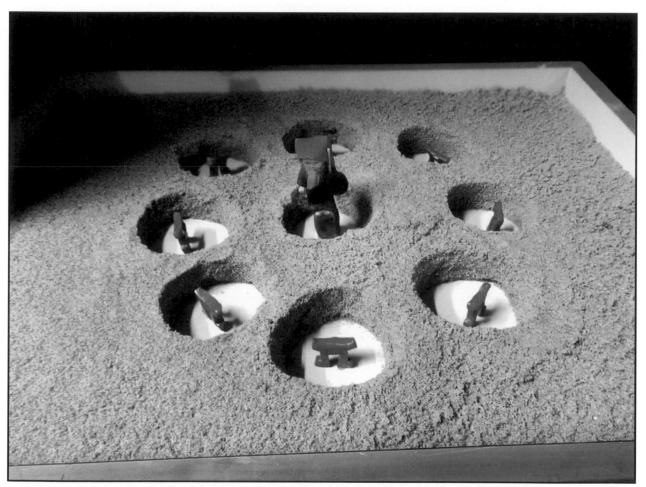

**Tray 14**
**Boy Age 15**

This is the Hero of Strasbourg. Now he chooses a European hero. The chimney sweep cleans what has been made black by the fire. This one is a hero. So the fire can burn well. They are rakish, sexual figures.

The toriis are the entrance gates to holy places. Here in the center is a man on a piece of wood. Now he accepts a human life as his path and it is holy. The wood is solid and strong. We see that the tray combines the holiness of the toriis with the earthiness of the body.

There are eight toriis. Eight is the number of eternity. It is two times four. Four, according to Jung, is the totality. We think of the four corners of the world. Two times this may be even stronger. Eight is the micro-macrocosm. It is Kabalistic. The number nine is completion. The toriis sit on the water. He is in contact, at home with, the unconscious on many levels.

The chimney sweep is a black, dark figure. He carries a ladder, a bucket and brushes. It may be that he is still unconscious about this stage. This may indicate that this is still to come. Yet he feels something very valuable with all of the toriis. We can see how these divine qualities penetrate in all of these pictures. He is so humble in the center of the most divine.

D.T. Suzuki told me that they meditate for long hours in the monastery, but the body gets lazy. They have to clean the rooms and work in the afternoon. Without the physical activity, the mind gets lazy. It is very important that the children have tasks at home for a balance and a sense of belonging. Both mind and body need attention.

He made holes in the water here. Let's see what he reached down for and came up with.

# Tray 15
## Boy Age 15

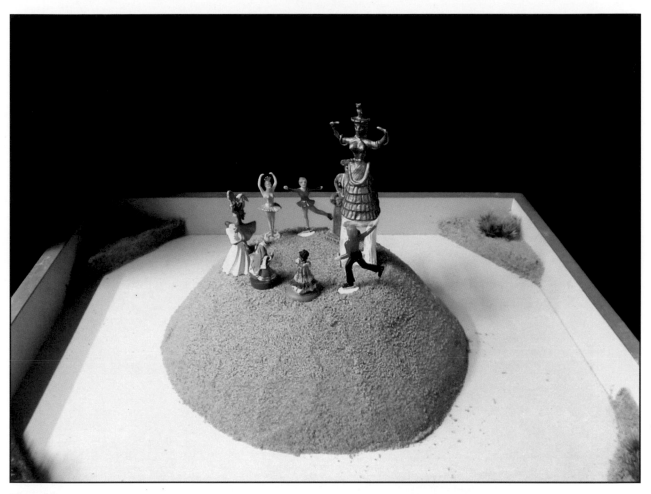

**Tray 15a**
**Boy Age 15**

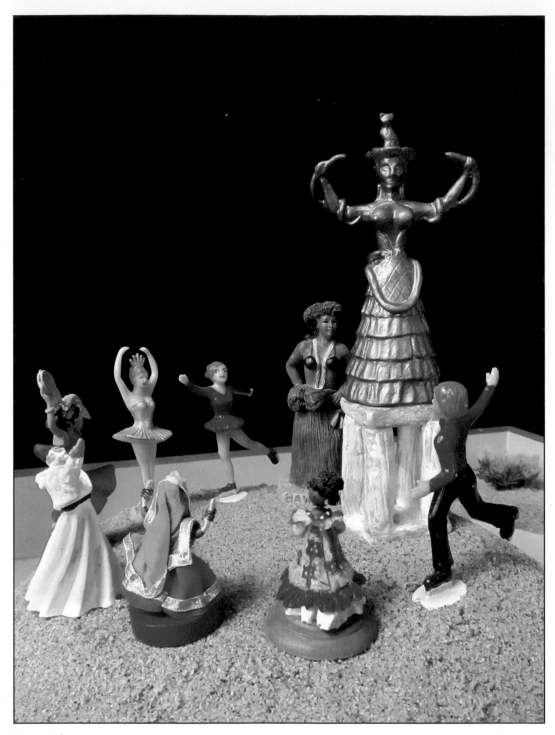

**Tray 15b**
**Boy Age 15**

*"This is the dance of the worship of the goddess of earth."*

He has a Greek temple, so he has reached back to the first tray now. There is dancing here – joy and a good feeling. This is a religious dance between earth and heaven. It is the movement of the body with music.

This looks like a birthday cake. This is a rebirth, a new birth. This is a festival for this goddess. Now he seems more anchored in artistic expression, and begins to feel more secure with it.

This is the Goddess of Crete. First he had to worship the chimney sweep, before worshiping the feminine. The goddess is higher, but they are all on the same island together. He really wanted her to stand inside the temple, but she was too big to go in there. He put her on top of the temple. Had she been inside, she would have been on the same plane with the dancers.

This temple is square. This is a symbol of earth and the earth is feminine. I would not think of this as feminine or masculine; it is an area. The Goddess of Crete was the last time the feminine was honored before the patriarchy. Her breast is bared. She had great courage. This is the feminine that can take on life, play with it and not be overcome by it.

Tray 16
Boy Age 15

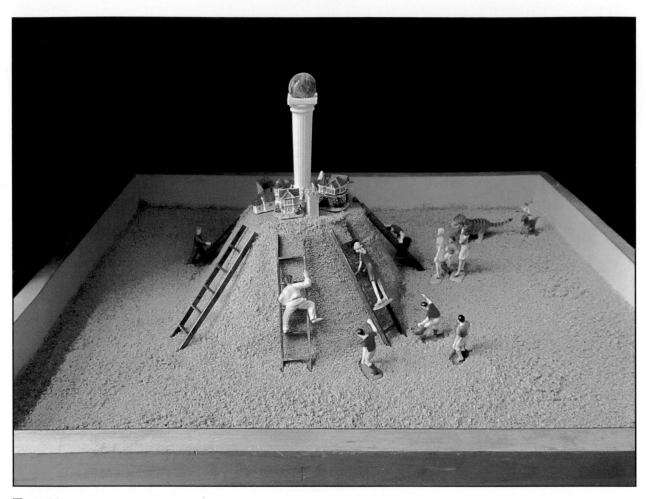

Tray 16a
Boy Age 15

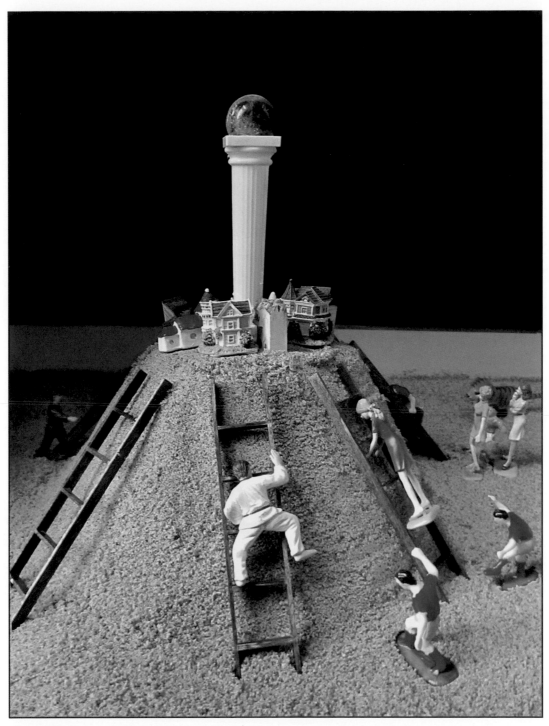

**Tray 16b**
**Boy Age 15**

Everyone is on the move to the center. They all want to get to the crystal ball. Animals and people are together here, looking toward the light, the crystal. This is much more conscious now. He sees that everyone is actually in need of the center, in need of this light. This shows how deeply he is affected by his work, because he wants everyone to do this. The city is now on the mountain with the light, in contrast with the separation of the city and the gods in the first tray.

The ladders make it accessible. In the past several trays he has had something up high that he wanted to reach. Inwardly he becomes religious. He experiences something deeply that helps him to develop. This is his trust. There is a lot of energy in this picture. He must apply this energy. This is his next task.

The process is never finished at the center. It is from this place that we must build up. It is hard for parents to leave the child in therapy past the manifestation of the Self, because they become so lively. They think all of the problems are gone. This is like the grass that comes out in Spring. It is tender and can be easily damaged. We have to bring the child up to where he really feels strong enough to deal with these energies. We have to find a place for these energies to be integrated and used.

It is uncomfortable that people have to climb up to the city to get the light. This is something that he as to put into action.

---

## Participant Question

*Should we ask the child where he is in the tray?*

Never ask if the child is here or there in a tray. What would this bring us? These are unconscious manifestations. If I make this connection for them, it is too early. We have to let the whole thing grow. Nature is at work, but we have to trust that it takes place.

Adults would like to know what things mean, but they have to accept that I do not interpret. Synchronicity does not take place if I interpret and do the work for them.

---

**Tray 17
Boy Age 15
Final Tray**

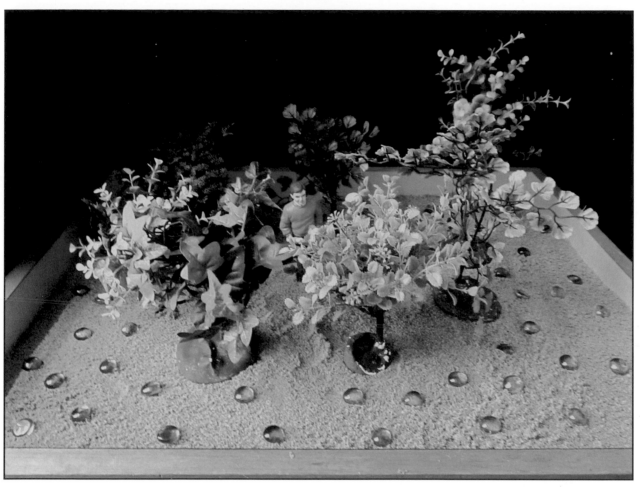

**Tray 17a
Boy Age 15**

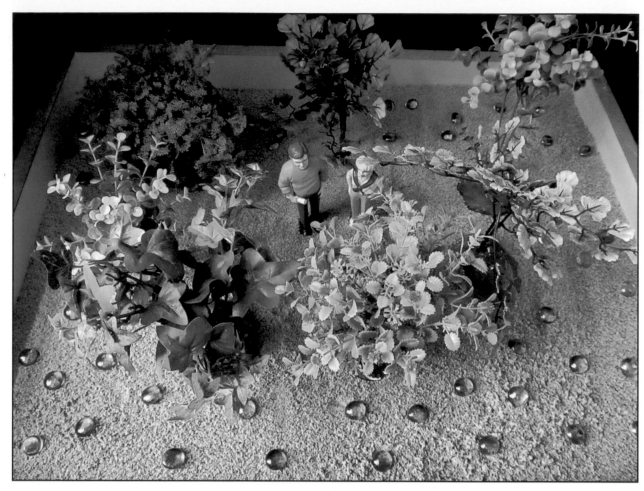

**Tray 17b**
**Boy Age 15**

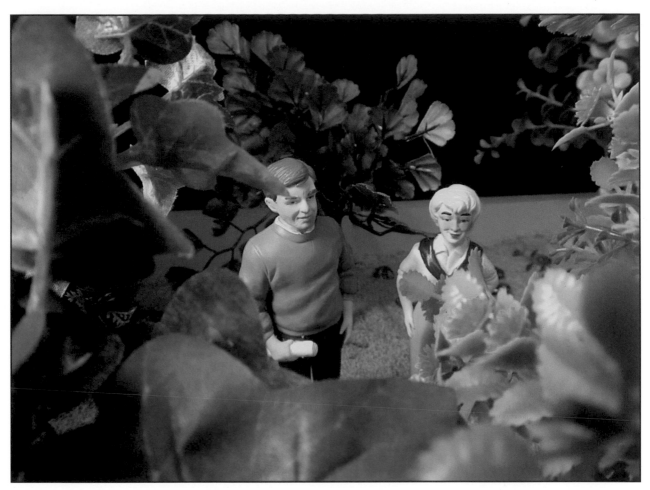

**Tray 17c**
**Boy Age 15**

This is his final tray. Here man and woman are together in the center of the jeweled firmament. He has found a friend. He is now with a friend in the earth, surrounded with the jewels of the heavens. He has found peace.

## *Participant Question*

*What are the differences between the wet and dry sand?*

Wet sand is easy to mold. Dry sand is difficult to mold. There are some resistances to wet sand, because it may be cold. This can have a deeper meaning. These are people who do not want to enter the unconscious, or who have resistance. Wet sand is the water and the earth. Dry sand is more delicate. You always have to see the person, the circumstances and where they are. We cannot give rules about this. We must be observant and understanding.

Sometimes psycho-somatic patients use the dry sand. I have worked with many patients with intestinal diseases – ulcers, colitis, and so on. These people prefer dry sand. Sometimes they prefer to just let the sand run through their fingers. They may not make any pictures. It is wrong to tell someone what we think they need to do. You can tell them, when it seems they want to, "You can put a tree, make a man coming," etc., but never say, "Make a sand picture." We can only give their inner life the opportunity where they are free to do what they want.

Pay attention when someone does not touch the sand - pay attention to what might come up from underneath. This may precipitate a psychotic break.

*What are the differences in the sandplay processes of adolescent boys and adolescent girls?*

Girls are also between the two worlds of childhood and adulthood, but the adult world of womanhood is different. The animal-vegetative level is the same for the girl as for the boy. But I do not see much of the fighting stage with girls. Girls will have horses. They want to ride a horse and to care for the horse. Maybe this is a "horse stage" for the girls. They come from the animal level into this level. This is the next step of development. First they care for the horse, and then they ride it. The caring for others follows this.

Sitting on a horse is the best situation for the body. It is absolutely in harmony in this position and the movement forward is very good for the body. The girls must feel very good in their bodies when they ride. They get in contact with their instincts. The girl learns to pay attention to the sensitivity of the horse. This is wonderful and should be introduced in the schools. When someone rides a horse, the back and organs are in absolute proper positions.

*How do we recognize the last tray?*

Very often it is clearly the last tray. Often the child will tell me, "Well, I am not coming next week." They know.

The man from this case went through school, through his *matura*, (the final exam upon finishing high school that must be passed in order to go on to the university.) He went abroad to study dance and music. Now he is studying filmmaking.

---

**End**
**Boy Age 15**

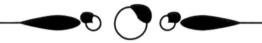

# Development Toward Pregnancy

*11th March 1988 - 2 Hour Lecture*

*San Francisco, California*

We are the only living creatures that are able to touch both earth and heaven. We must learn of this more consciously. The conscious and the unconscious have the capacity to bloom. Since the Middle Ages we have become more involved with the rational way of living and we forget about the other qualities. This is the masculine side. Many women are not aware that we are suffering from this. Today this is so significant that it may prevent women from becoming pregnant. The feminine quality is lost, thwarted.

There are so many possibilities for women today that they forget the main qualities that have been given to them by birth. This feminine quality has to do with love, compassion. This is not emotional love. We must try to bring this quality about. Out of this grows a spiritual quality, because this love is connected with the divine. It is actually this divine quality that belongs to the woman.

Sandplay is a medium through which we can touch this quality. The therapist must be fully able to accept what is coming from the client. This way the client can feel free and accepted. At this moment he is able to show the therapist, in the language of the sandplay, an entry into deeper realms within himself. There may be very dark elements here that prevent the blossoming of the flower. We do not stop here. We go deeper. Beyond the shadow, there is a spot that is clear, free and that is harmonious. This is the Self.

It is rare that this is achieved, but we have the possibility to go this deep. This is the original Self, which is given by birth. From here another personality can develop - a personality which is guided by the original Self. This is where one finds one's own potentials. Not those that belong to someone else.

With pregnancy we must see what is necessary to discover.

## Tray 1
## Development Toward Pregnancy

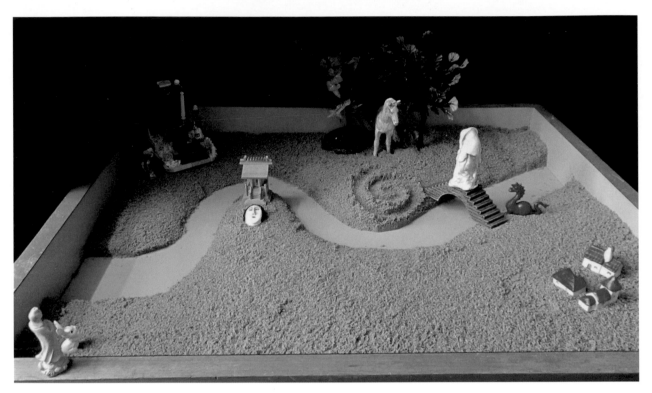

**Tray 1a**
**Development Toward Pregnancy**

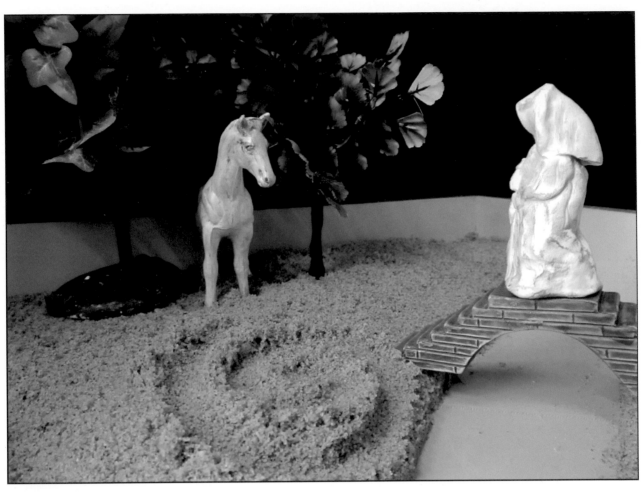

**Tray 1b**
**Development Toward Pregnancy**

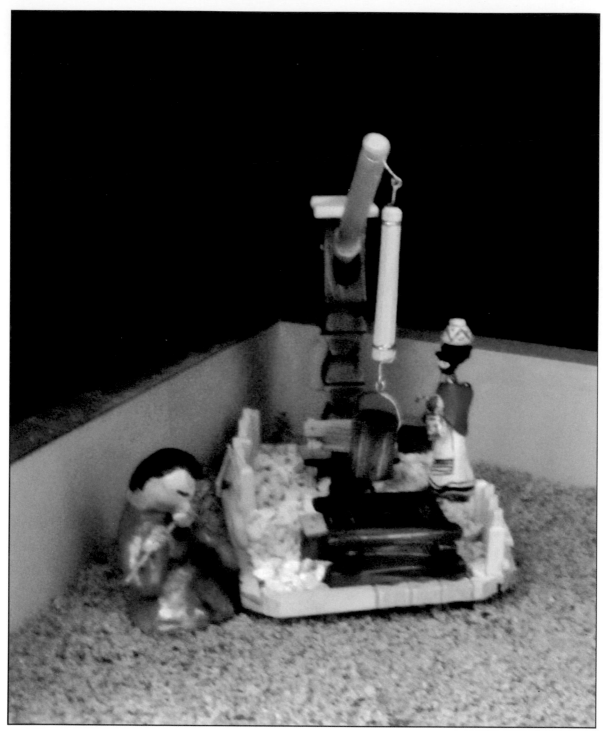

**Tray 1c**
**Development Toward Pregnancy**

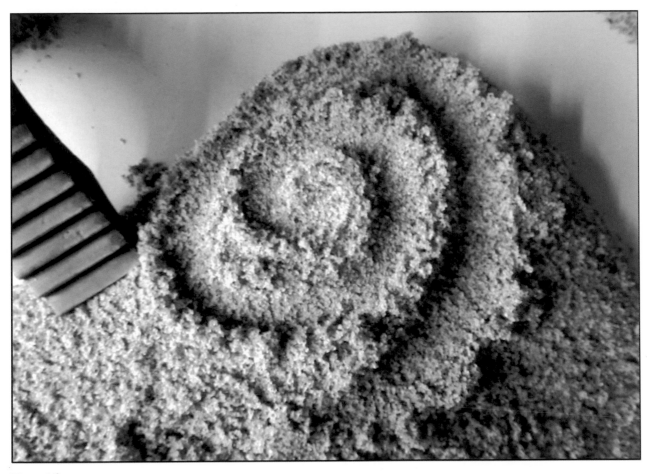

**Tray 1d**
**Development Toward Pregnancy**

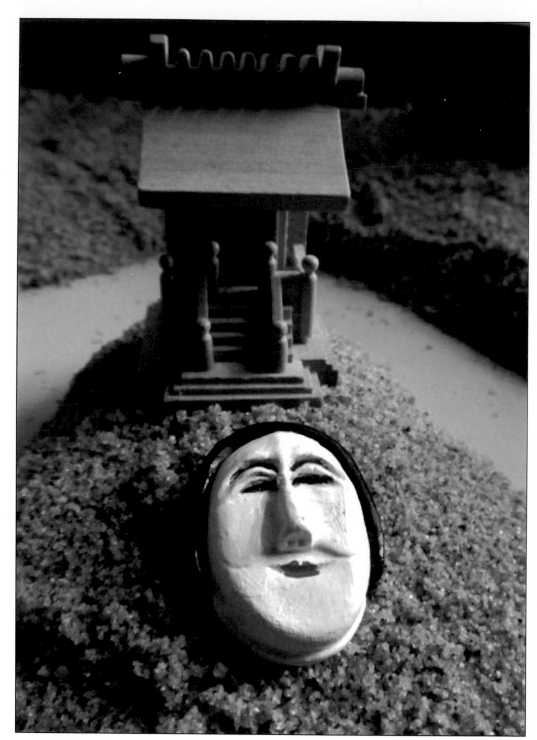

**Tray 1e**
**Development Toward Pregnancy**

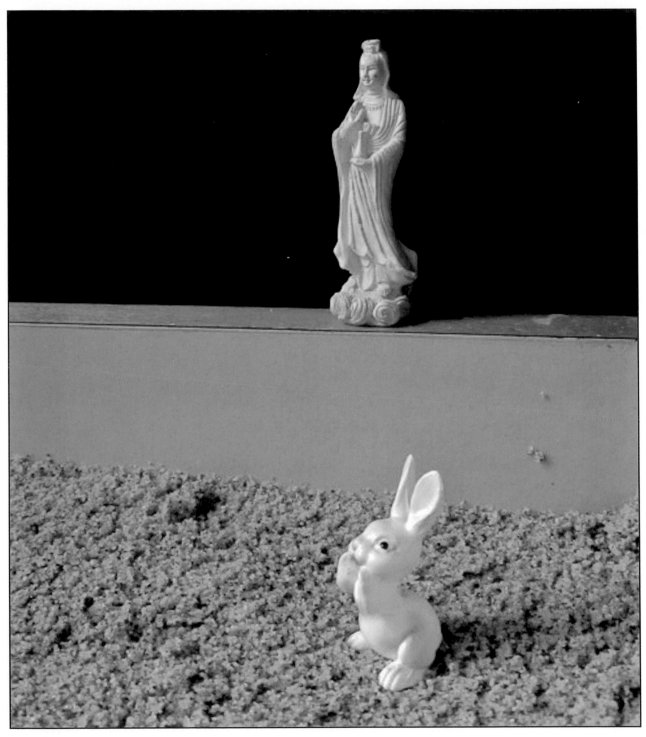

**Tray 1f**
**Development Toward Pregnancy**

The city is barren. The dragon may be furious. Red is about feeling and love, but when it has not been able to develop it can become aggressive.

The bride is beginning a new life. (Crossing the bridge) She will cross the river and encounter the spiral. The spiral is a development from within to the outer. Here it points to the white horse.

The white horse has a divine quality. Jesus is on a white horse in the apocalypse. Mohammed rides a white horse, and in China, white horses are kept in temples. This is about a divine instinct, and it is not yet a person.

The horse stands between two trees which are nature. The nature of this person contains this developing quality on an instinctual level, which may not be conscious.

The well is where we can get water from the depths. This may mean that there is a content in the unconscious, which can be brought up to consciousness. This will be the feminine nature that is connected with the masculine side and with art and music. The dark woman may be the unconscious side within herself which has a baby.

The white rabbit has the capacity to transcend during life. Buddha was a rabbit in a former incarnation.

Kwan Yin is the goddess of great compassion. This is the love for one's neighbor.

This mask is from the Noh theater - a philosophical, religious theater. The beauty of the young woman (mask) indicates the real capacity for the woman to be beautiful. This is connected to the temple, and thus to the divine.

Often the first tray will show the cause, the path of the therapy and the solution. It is up to the therapist to understand this language.

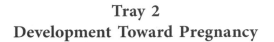

Tray 2
Development Toward Pregnancy

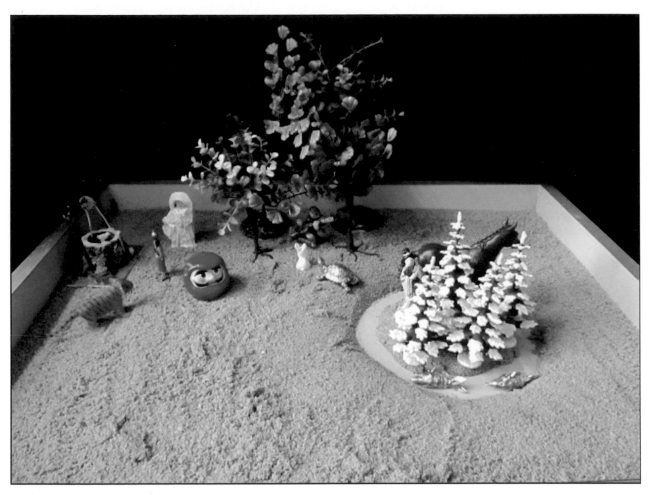

Tray 2a
Development Toward Pregnancy

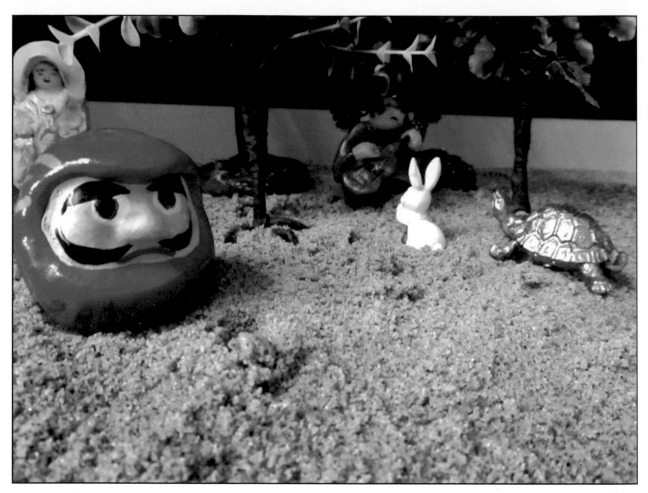

**Tray 2b**
**Development Toward Pregnancy**

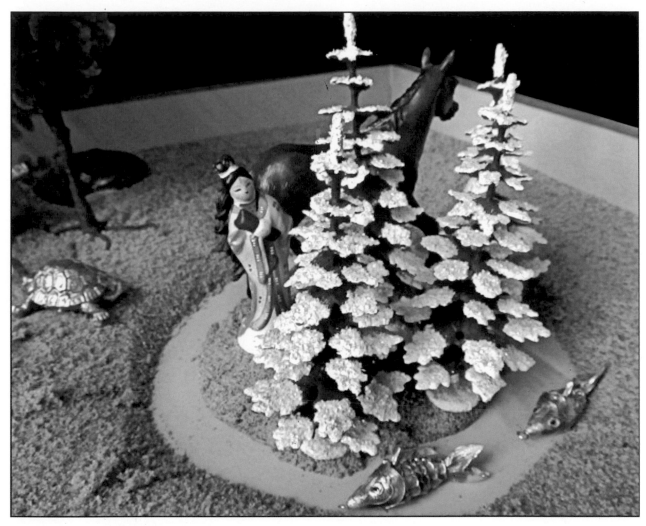

**Tray 2c**
**Development Toward Pregnancy**

The turtle contains the masculine and the feminine, the heaven and the earth. The heaven is the round shell on the back. Underneath is the square shell, the earth.

The man with the guitar is a masculine side that will be developed with an artistic quality.

The rabbit is feminine.

The Bodhidharma had great patience. Great patience is required to achieve what is indicated here.

The Japanese bride wears a white headdress to cover any horns of jealousy.

The tiger is wild and aggressive, especially when hungry. There may be some untamed negative energies displayed here that may need to be transformed.

The red flower is a blooming of her feeling function. She feels instinctively that this can be developed.

## Tray 3
## Development Toward Pregnancy

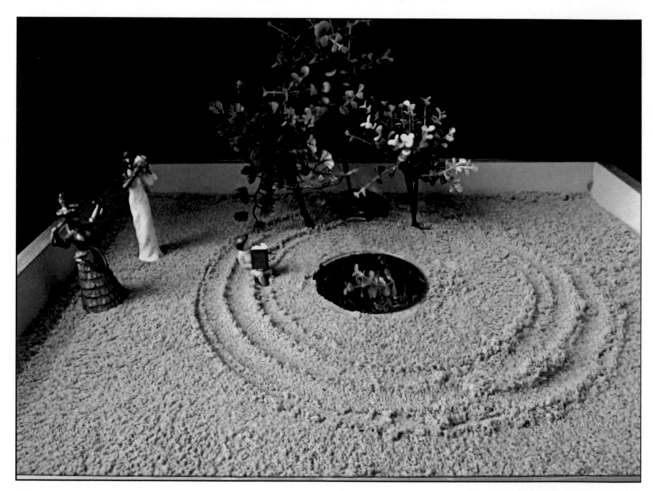

**Tray 3a**
**Development Toward Pregnancy**

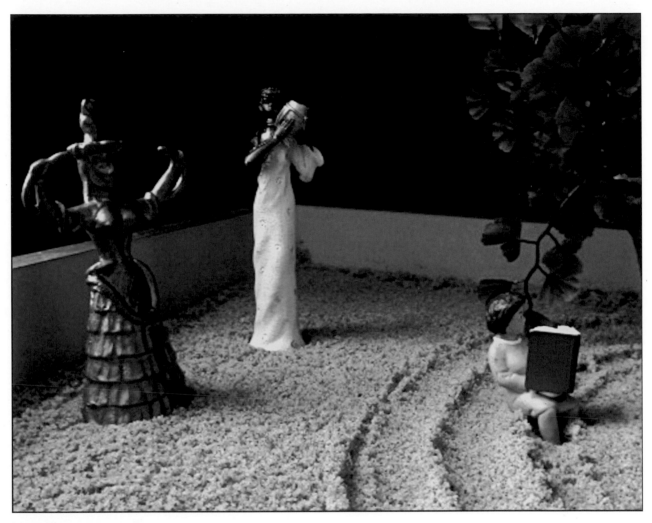

**Tray 3b**
**Development Toward Pregnancy**

Many things sit around the woman with the book. They have no relationship to her, because she is reading and is not interested.

The snake goddess of Crete is the feminine quality that is waiting, while the woman in the center is not in tune with her.

**Tray 4**
**Development Toward Pregnancy**

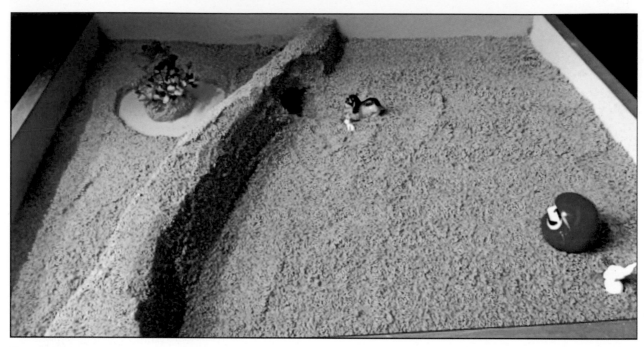

**Tray 4a**
**Development Toward Pregnancy**

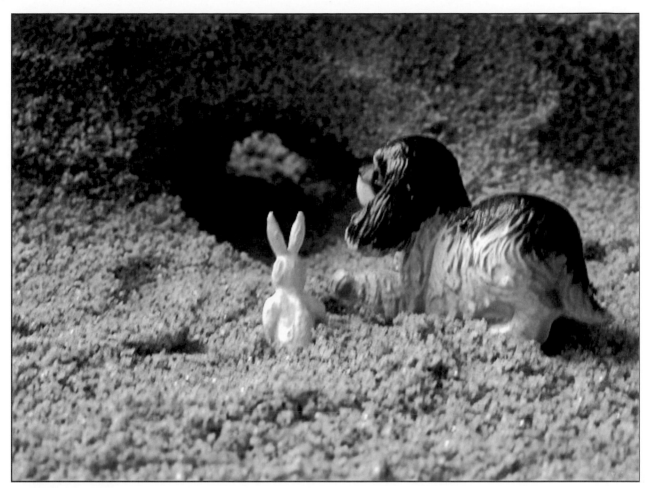

**Tray 4b**
**Development Toward Pregnancy**

There is a wall between two sides, but there is a possibility to reach the other side through a tunnel. She has to go to deeper levels of the unconscious to reach this.

The red color becomes something to be achieved.

The dog and the rabbit are animals, instincts. She will have to penetrate within herself to reach the instinctual levels to attain what is hidden.

## Tray 5
## Development Toward Pregnancy

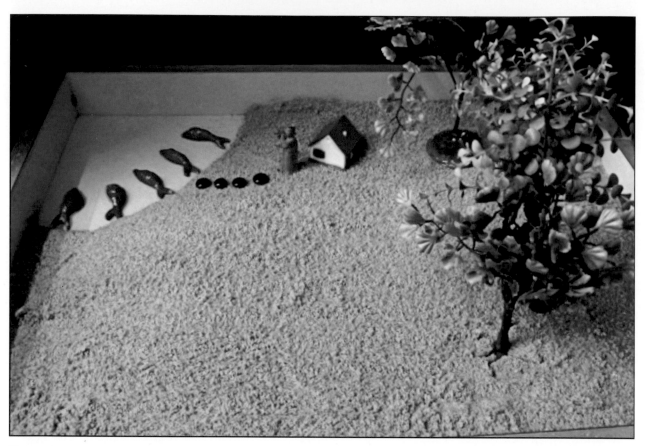

**Tray 5a**

**Development Toward Pregnancy**

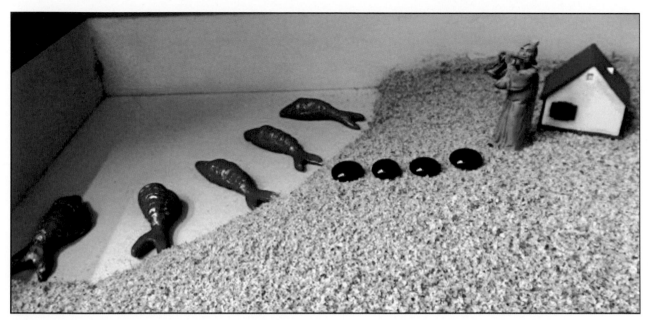

**Tray 5b**
**Development Toward Pregnancy**

Red becomes more important as she comes closer to the feeling function.

## Tray 6
## Development Toward Pregnancy

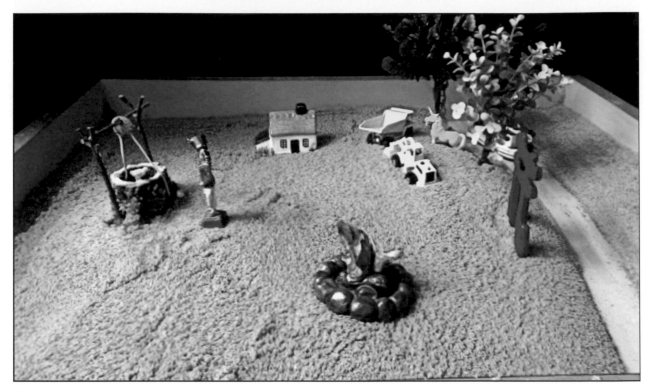

**Tray 6a**

**Development Toward Pregnancy**

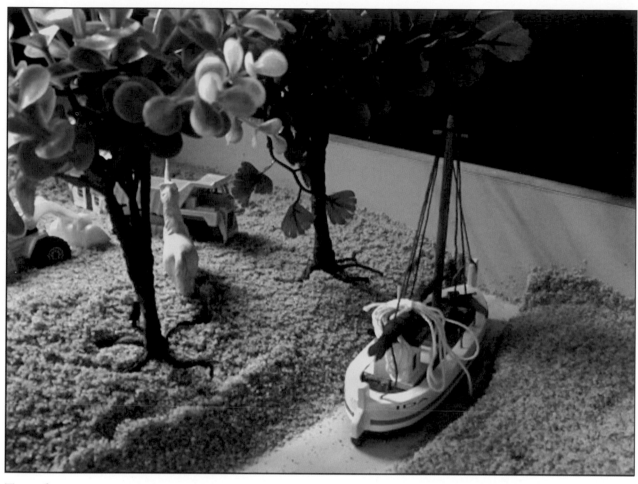

**Tray 6b**
**Development Toward Pregnancy**

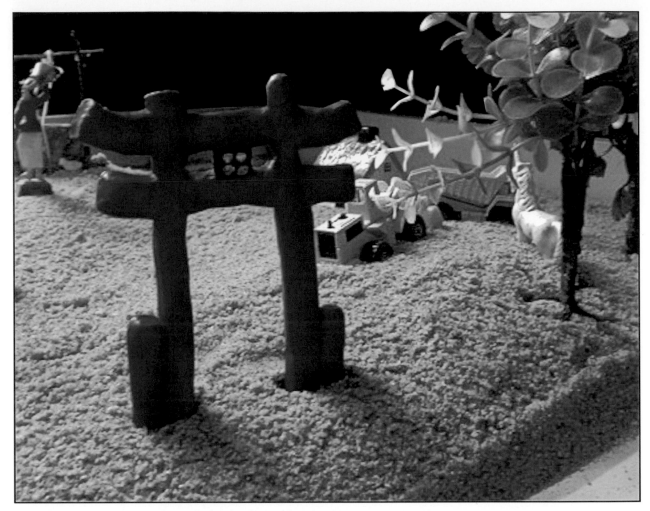

**Tray 6c**
**Development Toward Pregnancy**

Here is the torii. The divine begins to emerge. When we see Japanese figures in a Western person's tray, we can say that we are going very deep into the unconscious.

Here there is fire, water and earth, the three basic elements of the body. A fourth element is air, and the fifth may be the spiritual level.

The unicorn has to do with access to the spiritual. The two horns are bound together as one. All of the elements are displayed here. This shows the total aspect of this person. No wonder there is a torii here. When the elements are in harmony, the person is healthy. We look for an indication that all elements are equally developed, so they can play together.

The boat seems to be on the way to somewhere else.

## Tray 7
## Development Toward Pregnancy

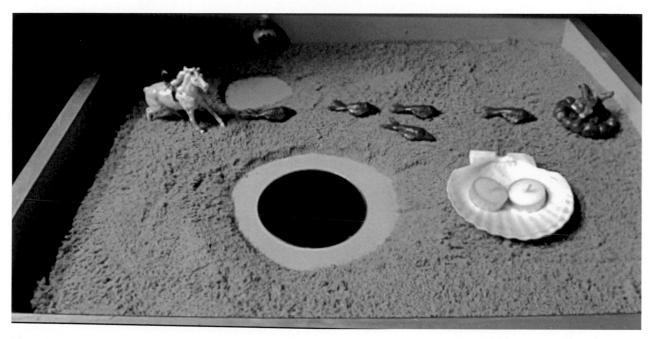

**Tray 7a**
**Development Toward Pregnancy**

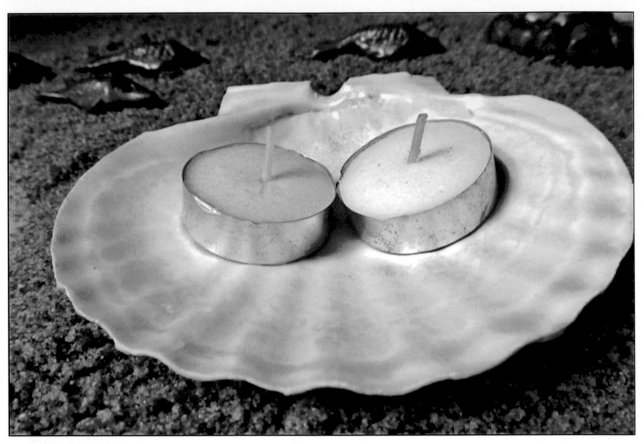

**Tray 7b**
**Development Toward Pregnancy**

The vessel is the feminine quality.

These fish are out of water.

The mirror indicates that she is slowly becoming more conscious of what is going on.

The two candles in the shell are not lighted. There is still some time before we can see a pure development. But there is an indication toward the fire.

### Tray 8
### Development Toward Pregnancy

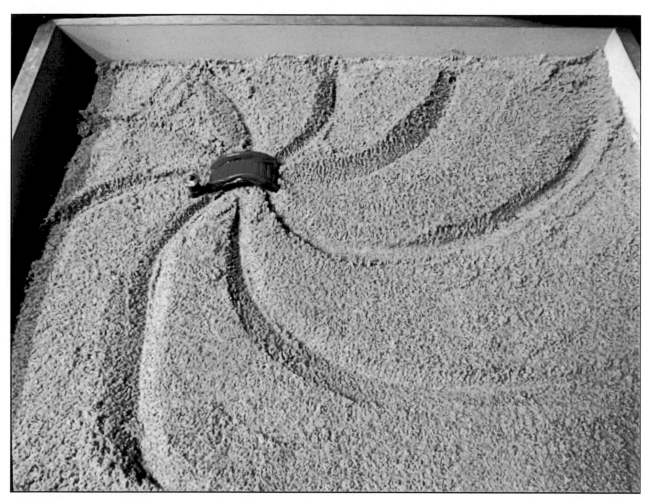

**Tray 8a**
**Development Toward Pregnancy**

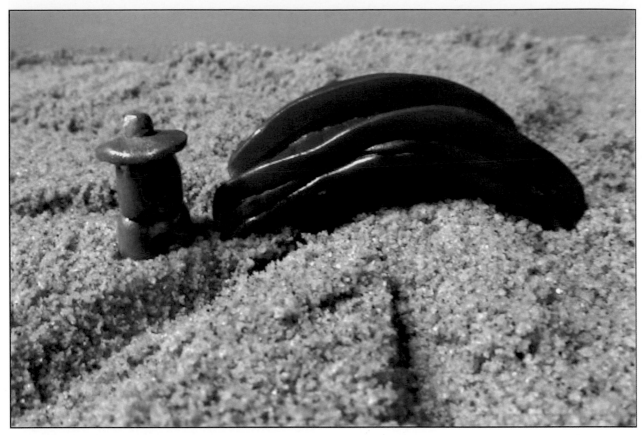

**Tray 8b**
**Development Toward Pregnancy**

This is the manifestation of the Self. The bridge brings the two sides together.

The wheel usually means that there is some light coming into the person. This is an image of the total aspect of the personality. The lantern is a light. From one light inside (the lantern) it reaches other elements. Here we come to a point where a transformation of energies can take place. At the manifestation of the Self there is a possibility for destructive energies to become constructive and positive.

## Tray 9
## Development Toward Pregnancy

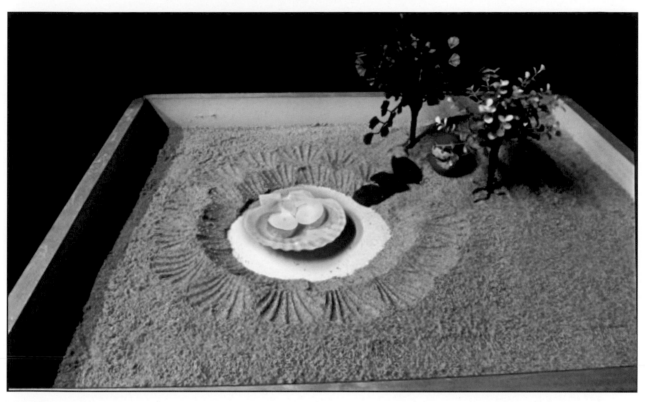

**Tray 9a**

**Development Toward Pregnancy**

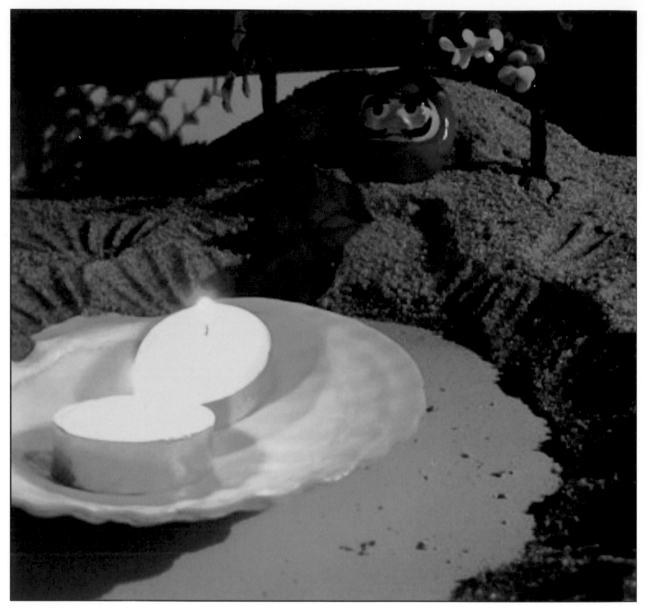

**Tray 9b**
**Development Toward Pregnancy**

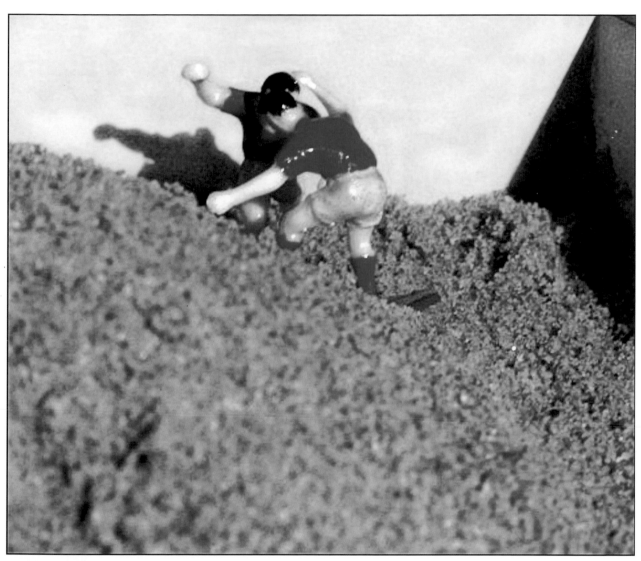

**Tray 9c**
**Development Toward Pregnancy**

The candles are lit. There is light and it is warmer. The shell imprints are the pure feminine quality. In the middle of this there is now light and warmth.

There is a fight going on. The transformation cannot take place fully yet. The Bodhidharma looks toward the light. He is patient and knows that the fight may be over later on. He sits between two trees, indicating that this is a natural way of development.

## Tray 10
## Development Toward Pregnancy

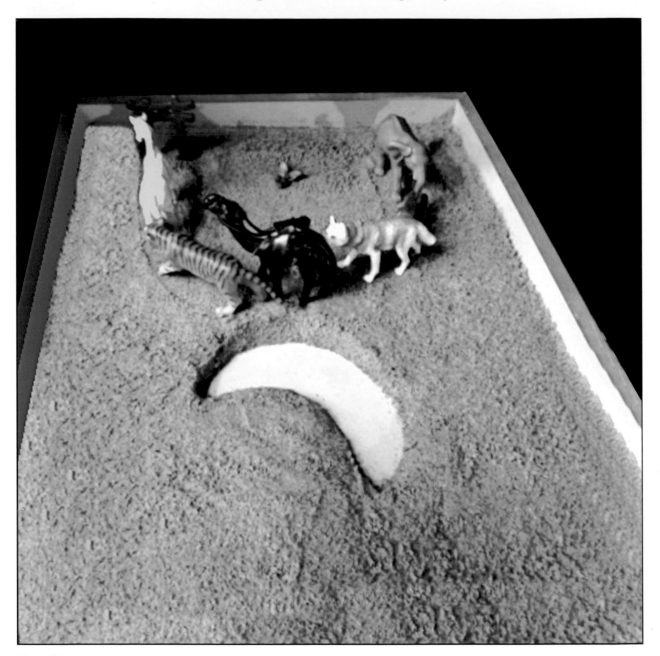

**Tray 10a**
**Development Toward Pregnancy**

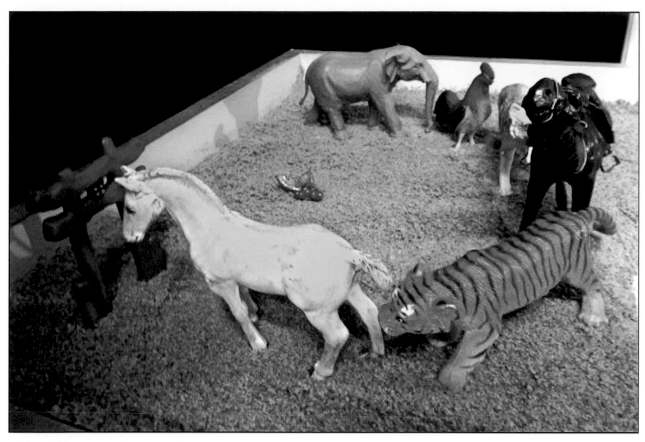

**Tray 10b**
**Development Toward Pregnancy**

The white horse guides all of the animals to drink and to go toward the torii. The guidance of the white horse has to do with getting in touch with the instinctual level of the divine quality.

The crescent-shaped lake is like the crescent moon. This is feminine. Here the instincts bring the feminine and the divine together. This is very important, because this was less developed at the beginning.

There are red berries. Red has appeared in every tray. The feminine and the divine come together here.

## Tray 11
## Development Toward Pregnancy

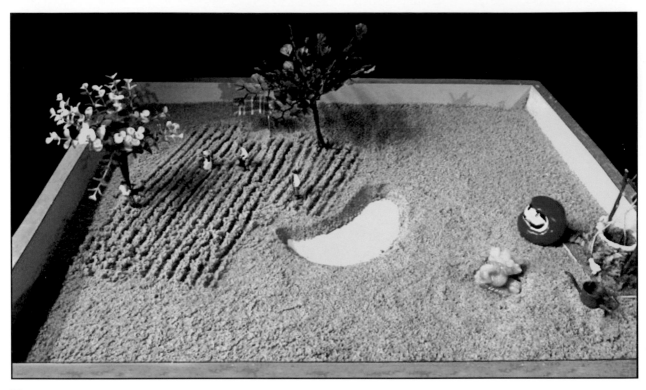

**Tray 11a**
**Development Toward Pregnancy**

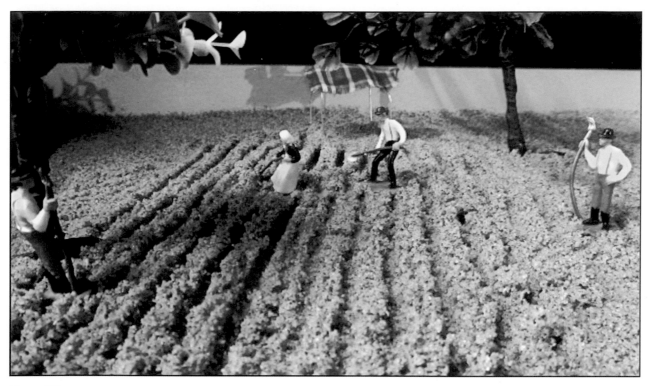

**Tray 11b**
**Development Toward Pregnancy**

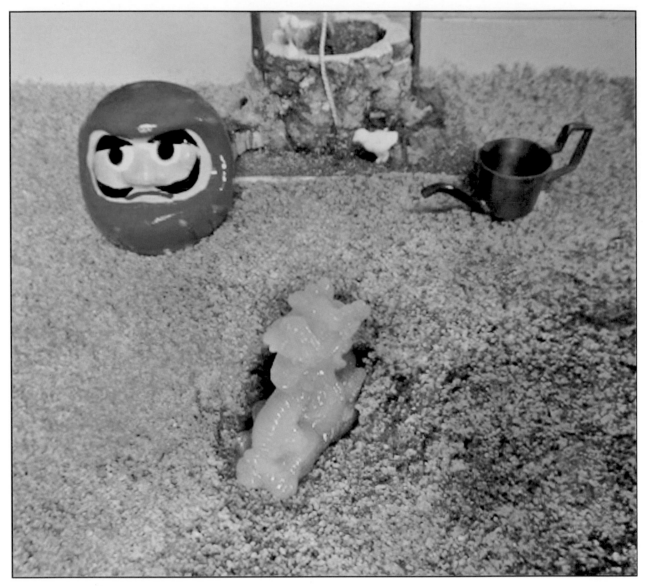

**Tray 11c**
**Development Toward Pregnancy**

Water is being fetched from the depths. Now it is time to be active with this. Before it was just potential.

The green dragon comes out of the cave. This is Spring, new life comes out of the earth. It is now completely in tune with nature and new life.

The farmers are working. They begin a new activity that is in tune with the earth.

## Tray 12
## Development Toward Pregnancy

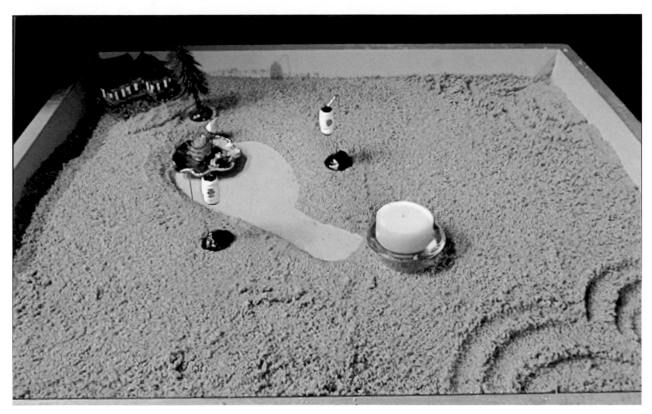

**Tray 12a**

**Development Toward Pregnancy**

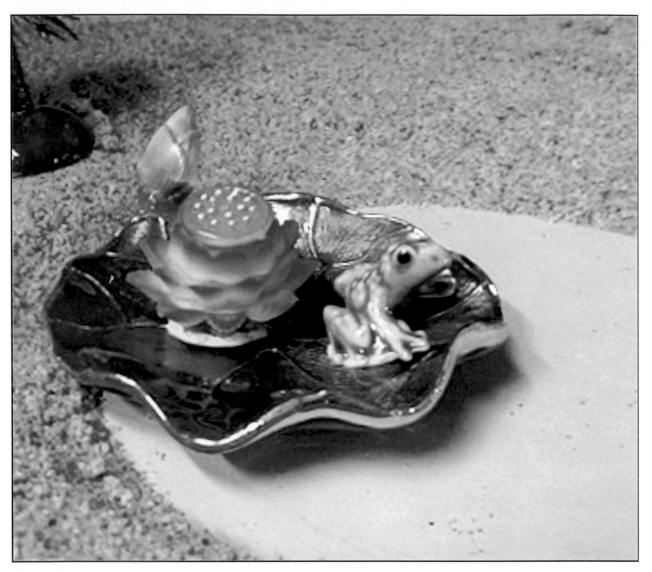

**Tray 12b**
**Development Toward Pregnancy**

The green frog on the lotus is next to the Self. The lotus is the birth of a divinity. This is one of many times a lady became pregnant after using the frog on the lotus leaf. This is the divine quality of the experience of birth. Birth is a divine happening. This is the right way to express this – to receive a child as God's gift. This tray indicates that this may happen. The water way looks like a uterus and birth canal. The tree is natural growth. In Japan the frogs play a big role, because they live in the water and sit on the leaves of the lotus. They have closeness to the divine.

## *Participant Questions*

*Can you tell us about the meanings of the four quadrants of the tray?*

I do not like to do this, because the sandplay is three-dimensional. This can be done with a painting, however. The sandplay work penetrates into the archetypal world, rather than the ego world. So symbols of this world come up. To do sandplay you must understand what is going on and you must undergo the same process. This is hard work.

*Why is it that you do not interpret the sandplay?*

When an inner happening corresponds with an outer happening, this is the resolution and the person is ready to go to the next step. The images anticipate events to come. It takes time to bring this up from an unconscious level to a conscious level. If you try to explain right away, this would force an interpretation before the person was ready for it. We damage the process when we interpret too soon. Explain to your client that you do not interpret and why.

*What do you tell the person to do when they come to your office?*

I say, "Hello. How are you? What would you like to do today?"

**End
Development Toward Pregnancy**

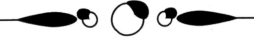

# Sandplay in Switzerland

*25th July - 12th August 1988*

*Zollikon, Switzerland*

The soul has its secret ways. We will know more if we concentrate on the soul.

During this course we will see three cases: one of a child, an adolescent and an adult.

There is one main issue in the work with sandplay. It happens on a very deep level. With this tool we have access to the deepest layers within ourselves and the deeper unconscious. Why does this happen? My whole psychology is based on a free and protected space. It is the task of the therapist to provide such an environment. With the sand we work from a very deep level, a very deep transference.

I have encountered the deepest work in Japan, where the deep transference is common in daily life. Without speaking, the Japanese understand what is going on with the next person. They make a connection on a deep level. Each knows what the other is feeling without talking about it. They all participate in what is going on inside themselves and with the other people. If they stay away from each other they lose contact. This is why they do not take long holidays.

Sandplay was first accepted in Japan. This is likely because I told them that I do not explain what is going on in the process. They can just experience what is brought up. Not all of you will be able to do this, but I would like to show you. This is about seeing the Self, the aspect of the total psyche of our being with all of its tremendous secret knowledge. We have access to so much if we get in touch with this. This is a wisdom, an inner wisdom.

We aim to touch this layer. It is very valuable. We cannot demand to see this in a person. I have to be free of wanting to see it in the other. I must be completely free to allow whatever wants to happen from within. This free space is very important.

What is a free space? This is a place where there is unconditional love and no judgment. It is not easy to provide this. Things come across that we do not like. We have to ask, *"Do you really allow this, or just act as if you do?"* Sometimes it is seen as a weakness to just be there, but it takes a lot of energy, understanding, and presence. The more we are able to provide such a space, the better the clients are able to display whatever comes up with them. There may be weakness or danger – then comes the second part. We have to protect them from going beyond their limits. We have to be very sensitive to know this. On one side we have to be free; on the other side we must protect them from danger. If you see that there is a possibility of a psychotic break, do not continue with sandplay. Sandplay activates the unconscious so much that we must be able to see when a sandplay is in a safe place and when it is not. I do not tell the client but I see that they are trembling, etc. Next time they come I just talk with them, not about the danger, but about them, slowly preparing the ground for another sandplay. They will tell you when it is time.

I ask the client if they would like to do a sandplay, but they have to decide themselves. I never tell them to do a sandplay. Something within them tells them. They know what is going on.

I always talk with the person first. I tell them about sandplay, that we can do dream analysis, that we can always talk. If they appear to be having difficulties I can say, *"I see we are maybe a little stuck. Maybe we can try something else."*

We tell them that the talking does not gain so much, but that there is another possibility in the sand. I tell the client that the sand is something different that we do not come across in our daily lives. I tell them that it is play and it has its own special qualities. I have to take away their idea that I just want to make them small like a child. Friedrich Schiller said that the human being is only complete when he can play.

I tell the client that we do have rules: the sand box is of a certain size, which we do not go beyond. You can move the sand, form it or run it through the fingers. Between the freedom and the rules, the limitations, there is the completeness. The human being is always dealing with these opposites: light – dark; freedom – limitation. The aim is always to be more complete, more whole. We must remember this. Through play we fulfill the need to become more complete.

To provide this space, you must have this aim yourself. We can never stop with our inner work. Doing this work makes us small and humble. If we are truly like this and think that maybe we can help a little bit, we can have a better attitude. This is the opposite of the values in our world now. Every day I go to work saying I will let myself be surprised. If I expect something it will not happen. If I am open and respectful of each person, we've already taken a big step.

## Friedrich Schiller's References to Play

Friedrich Schiller's poetry is filled with references to play.
This concluding stanza from his work, *Thekla: A Spirit Voice*, is a beautiful example:

> Faith is kept in those blest regions yonder
> With the feelings true that ne'er decay.
> Venture thou to dream, then, and to wander
> Noblest thoughts oft lie in childlike play.

*Thekla, 156-7*
*Poems of the Third Period, by Friedrich Schiller*

# Boy Age 12
# Failed Exams

A twelve year-old boy has failed his exams and his parents are upset.

## Tray 1
## Boy Age 12

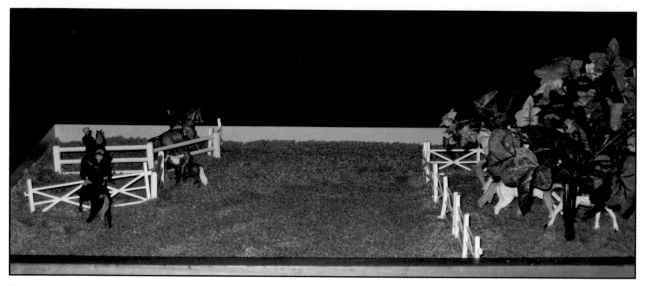

**Tray 1a**
**Boy Age 12**

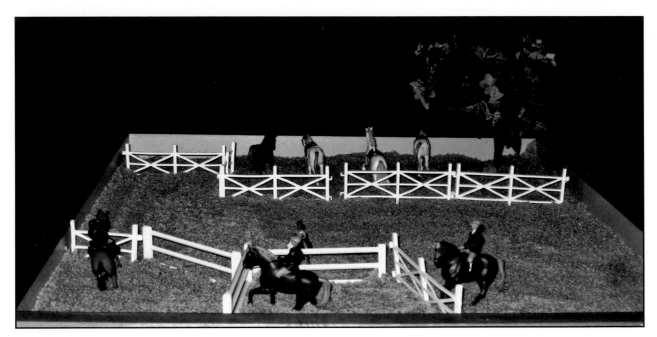

**Tray 1b**
**Boy Age 12**

*It is a training place to learn to ride horses.*

The first thing you do is to be aware of your first impression. Here the left side is two thirds of the tray. It predominates. The hurdles are very constrained and there is not enough space for the horses to jump. It is very difficult.

The right side is more restful. He is taking the hurdles, but from a contained space. Maybe this tells us how he has to take the hurdles - without any real preparation. He is forced to do something and it takes up a lot of space – two thirds of his life. There is some leisure, so we see that it is not all difficult.

The horse represents energy. It is instinctual, pure instinct; he knows the way. The horse gets frightened easily, but is very powerful.

With animals in the sand trays, look into their behaviors in nature. These represent behaviors within us, our instincts. The horse is mystical because it knows its way in the dark.

In this tray there are three brown horses exercising, and one brown and three white on the leisure side. The brown have an active, instinctual energy.

The white horse has a divine quality. We see this in Buddhism, Christianity and Islam. In Christianity in the apocalypse there are four riders on four different colored horses: white, red, yellow and dark. The rider on the white is said to be Christ. In Buddhism there is a story of a monk who rode to India on a white horse to gain knowledge. (*The Journey to the West*) In Japan white horses are kept in the temples. The Dali Llama was offered a white horse to travel from Tibet to India that he might ride safely. In Islam, the prophet Mohammed rode to heaven on a white, winged horse after his death.

Because there are so many horses in this tray, it may be that there is some question about religion. The boy called some of them "Mexican." Why? The Mexicans are freer, more open, active than the stern Swiss. The boy's training, or schooling, is to jump the hurdles, maybe his exams. But he did not pass. Maybe the Mexicans represent the rest, the leisure that he needs. We over-regiment kids and ourselves. We have a hard time taking it easy.

This is his first tray. Is he under strain that he has to exercise to jump the hurdles? Does he need some rest? Is there a religious question? We do not know. We cannot tell for sure what he is going to see. We must learn to accept that we do not get a clear-cut picture of what is going on. We have to keep it all in mind. We have to wait, but without expectations.

## The Journey to the West

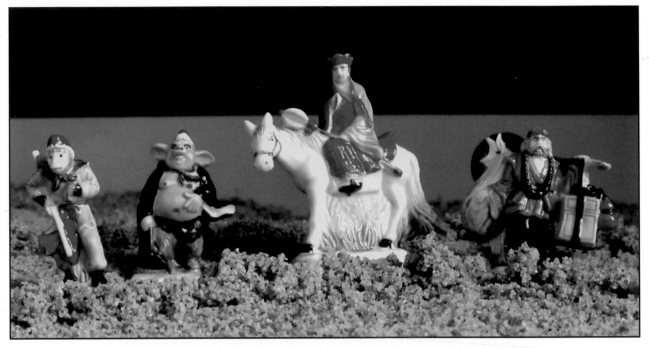

**Monkey, Pigsy, Xuan Zang and Sandy on their Journey**

The *Journey to the West* is among the great classic tales of Chinese literature, written by scholar, Wu Ch'eng-en in the late sixteenth century. It was abridged and translated into English by Arthur Waley in 1942, and re-named *Monkey*.

The *Journey to the West* recounts the well-known story of monk, Xuan Zang (602-664), whom Buddha appointed to travel to India to acquire the Buddhist scriptures for translation into Chinese. His journey becomes a colorful adventure during which he meets the main character, Sun Wukong, a monkey king with a colorful and rebellious past. Sun Wukong's name means *awakened to emptiness*. Born from a stone, he developed remarkable powers and strengths through his Taoist practices, which enabled him to defeat the many monsters and demons they encountered in their journey. Along the way, Xuan Zang and Sun Wukong are joined by Zhu Bajie (Pigsy in English) and Sha Wujing, (Sandy), both sent by the Buddha to serve as helpers. Sha Wujing is a man whose name translates as *sand awakened to purity*, and Zhu Bajie's name means *pig that rises to power*.

The story is arranged in three primary sections, including: the history of the Monkey King, Sun Wukong; the story of the monk, Xuan Zang before he set out upon his sacred journey; and the many trials the group encounters along the way.

---

**Tray 2**
**Boy Age 12**

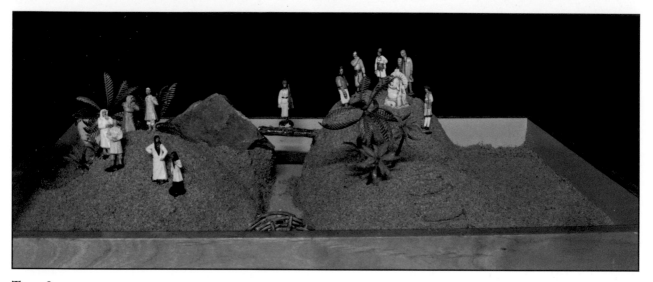

**Tray 2**
**Boy Age 12**

*This is a crossing of countries.*

This is the coming together of two different countries. He said that one belongs to the Indians and one to the Arabs. *"They have different religions and are not permitted to come together."*

You see that we are already on a deeper level of the unconscious. The process itself penetrates into deeper levels of the psyche.

The East honors the feminine. In Islam, the masculine is more dominant. There are more rules for their daily lives. This compares with the exercise/rest dynamic of Tray 1. Now this is on a deeper level of the psyche. We touch the ground of the collective unconscious, as he has had no contact with Buddhism or Islam.

Something religious seems to be separated and cannot come together. I then learned that the parents were Catholic and Protestant. They had decided not to baptize the children so that they might choose later for themselves. This shows that such an intellectual decision of the parents does not correspond to the needs of the child. He needs this security to meet with the other. This is the guard in the tray.

He chooses two different religions here, but not two different Christian religions. The collective unconscious does its part in everything. Because he may have had an affinity to one more than the other (Protestantism or Catholicism) he chose these two religions. One is more dominating (Islam) and one is more about growing from within (Buddhism.) It cannot come together like this. Something has to happen.

Because he has said the same thing in two ways, he is telling us that this is really a problem. (Two trays with masculine and feminine differences: one rigid and demanding, the other growing from within and relaxed). What he is aiming at is the bridge, but here he cannot pass over it.

Palm trees make the connection between heaven and earth. Perhaps this is a bridge for him. This may be a natural bridge for him, one coming from nature.

So far this is a clear-cut image of difficulties in his inner situation. Very often school difficulties are dependent on the development of the child that has been deprived of coming to the Self. The Self is given by birth. During the first year, the Self is taken care of by the mother. When the baby begins to walk, he alienates from the mother and takes the Self with him. The Self should manifest in the individual between two to four or five years. This means that they begin to talk about total aspects, symbols of the total aspects. They draw circles. If the circle is not complete, there is no security. They may draw squares. The basic need of the human being is the need to become complete. If this is disturbed or prohibited, they develop a needy ego that needs to re-connect with the Self.

The relationship between the Self and the ego is the primary relationship. So it is two sides of the Self and the ego that need to come together, not only the exercise-rest and Islam-India. This can happen when the ego realizes that it is only a part of the Self.

We are looking for the manifestation of the Self where we lay the base for a new development. People usually come to us because they have a needy ego. People go into the darkness until there is a breakthrough to the manifestation of the Self. The manifestation of the Self becomes the basis for a transformation of energies. This is a very deep experience of the true Self and can help the people confront the darker aspects.

**Tray 3**
**Boy Age 12**

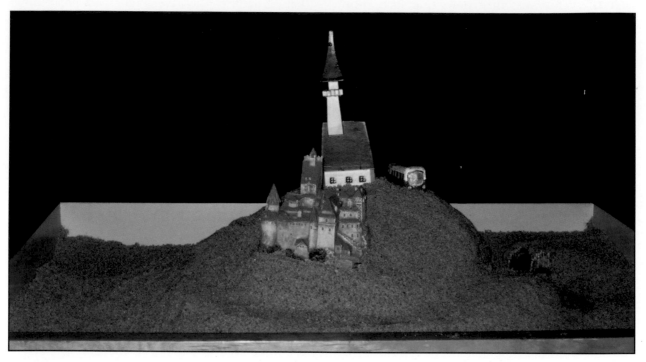

**Tray 3a**
**Boy Age 12**

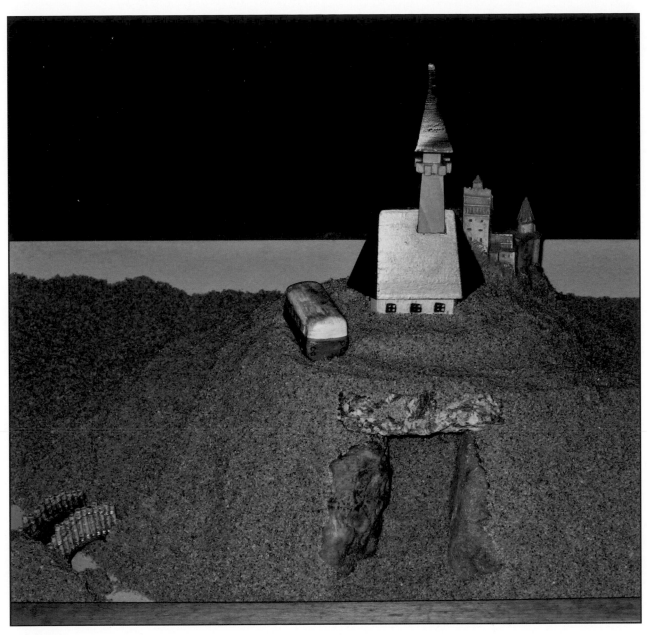

**Tray 3b**
**Boy Age 12**

*This is a place to come and see beautiful things.*

Notice that the bus is too big to cross this bridge. The tour bus is the observing aspect. The church is on the mountain and the castle is on the mountain. These are seen for their beauty, but not for the service that goes on inside.

When something is high up we need to compare it with the body. Something in the head is high up. This is something seen from a rational, intellectual way.

The church represents security. This is where we pray for health and protection. The castle is known to be a protected place. In this tray people go just to look at it.

On the back of the mountain he builds a cave with heavy stones. He says that he builds his own church. The church from the sight-seeing viewpoint does not provide the security. He needs his inner church and he builds it with large stones.

The cave is a womb. It has to do with being re-born. Something within him finds a re-birth. Here the two sides come together. Something new has to develop in this boy. This is what he was looking for, but consciously he has no idea of this.

This is something that we all need, this inner cave, inner spot where we will find security. It is from here that we can later deal with the outside world. Without this, the church becomes a sight-seeing place. And the castle, which used to protect us from outside attacks, also becomes a sight-seeing place.

He shows that the religion or security has nothing to do with the intellect, but with the inner most capacity. We all have this without exception. We just need to find it. With sandplay many people can find this inner security. We cannot provide this security, but can provide the free and protected space for the client to find their own inner security. He needed his own enrichment within himself.

**Tray 4**
**Boy Age 12**

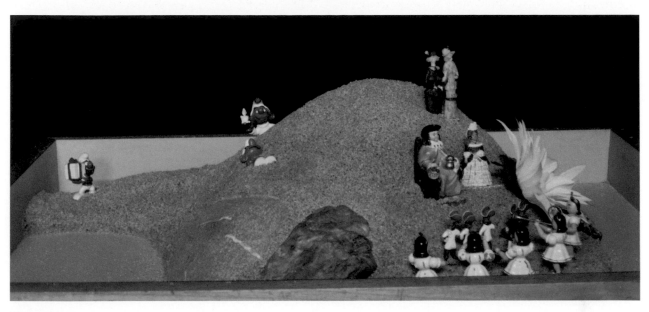

**Tray 4a**
**Boy Age 12**

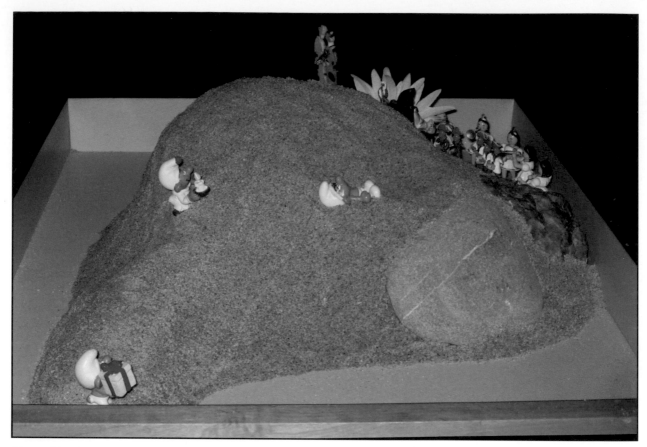

**Tray 4b**
**Boy Age 12**

He builds a strong hill with the stones he used to make a cave before.

The number two plays a big role here. Jung says that the number two in dreams indicates that this a problem that has to become conscious.

The king and queen are archetypes of leadership, of coming together.

He said that it was early in the morning, seven a.m., and they all come together. He thought that they all played an instrument and made an early morning concert. Here the feeling begins. Early in the morning is a new beginning.

He says, "*There are two old aunties and they complain about the noise.*" Maybe this points to the child's education. The old aunts are not open to his music. His education comes through here. The female education by the mother. Maybe she carries a masculine quality that is not in favor of the child's development. For a woman to complain about the music, this points to a negative animus quality in the mother. Two of them here means he experiences this very strongly.

In a way there is a chance that the two sides can come together. On the other side there is something preventing this. When a new element begins to break through, this movement is so tender and subtle. It is very easy for it to be destroyed again. It must be protected. The therapist must recognize when this begins to appear. Here he shows that there is a danger that it will be destroyed again.

There is a daisy here. Something begins to flower, to grow. The yellow center is the sun. The white is innocence, spirituality. As a central shape, this is the first indication of the Self. "Margarita" means "the pearl." This is a strong indicator for fine development. Here it comes out of the dark, on the side. This is why it is not yet a manifestation of the Self, but it is an indication that it is moving toward it. Something like this coming out of the side indicates that there will be a manifestation of the Self.

The two sides have not yet come together. This indicates that he has never experienced the manifestation of the Self, or it has happened, but has been thwarted through circumstances. We cannot tell for certain, but we can assume this. We do know that he has not had a good opportunity for strong development of the ego. Only when he is really nourished by the Self, when the two sides are together, then we can assume that there will be a healthy ego development. Here he suffers a needy ego.

I could see that my work in the sand corresponded with Neumann's notions of the development of the Self. He said, "*You are bringing me proof of my work.*" His work grew out of his research in myth, religion and literature. We were going to work together more, but he died shortly after. We never had the opportunity to discuss any further. But seeing this correspondence assured me that I should continue in this way.

What we see in this case is the need for another development of the ego. There is something that comes through the unconscious.

The Smurfs have pointed caps, which are images of bringing things into consciousness. They remind us of the dwarfs. They live in the darkness of the earth and appear in the night. They do all of the work for the dreamer. It could be that the Smurfs are modern dwarfs.

Smurfs were made in Germany. At the beginning I saw that they were all men. There was only one girl, who was a playgirl. I told the Germans that this represents the situation of Germany and they cannot estimate the true feminine. Now they have more females.

They are all blue. It could be a feminine color, because Mary is shown in a blue coat. Also the blue of the sky in sandplay. Jung said that blue was the thinking function. I think this applies here, because they activate the thinking function. Here this boy is in therapy because he is having trouble in school. This applies here. Maybe this is activating his thinking function. We always have to see what it could mean in this particular case. Smurfs also display many moods and many activities. I would call them many active energies coming up from the dark.

## Tray 5
## Boy Age 12

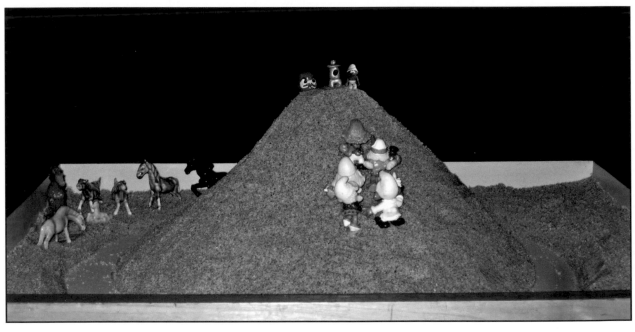

**Tray 5a**
**Boy Age 12**

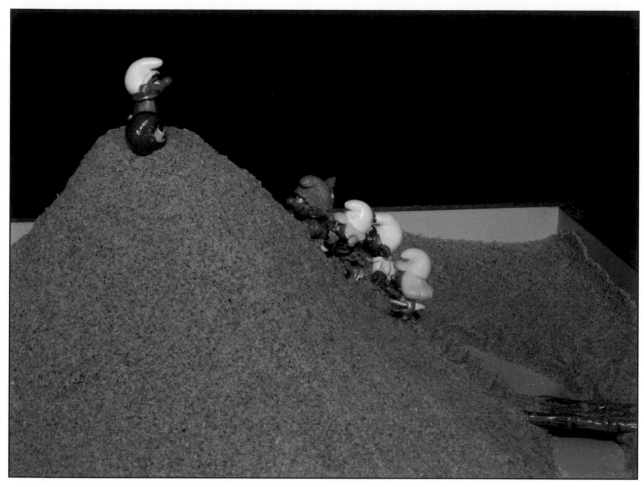

**Tray 5b**
**Boy Age 12**

Here he wanted to build a castle for the Smurfs. He said, "*This is a castle and there is someone with a trumpet in the morning at six a.m. When they blow it, everyone has to come outside of the castle.*" Early in the morning – it is an awakening, a new beginning.

This is a fortress. He builds a strong inner structure so he cannot be hurt anymore. Sometimes when I describe a needy ego, it is like an egg without its shell. When they build a strong fortress, it is the opposite. When he says, "*...at six a.m. everyone has to come outside,*" it could mean that now he is ready to come outside. Six a.m. is the dawn, the moment that the light comes.

In the first image the horses had to be trained. Here they are more at ease. They are colorful.

The Chinese porcelain horses are very beautiful and balanced. They are not saddled and are truly free to move. There are seven horses here. This may be associated with the seven gods, seven happy men, six masculine and one feminine.

Six a.m. is the time of the sunrise, the ending of the darkness. It is also two times three. Six is also the devil. We must see that there cannot be just pure light. There is always a dark side to things. There are the two sides he struggles with. This may have to do with this.

The three figures on the top of the hill are like a crucifixion.

The Bodhidharma has to do with patience. He waited many years for the Buddha to turn to him. When there is a tendency in sandplay for very fast development, we will see the Bodhidharma appear. It is as if he is saying, "…*wait a while; do not rush.*" We have to wait a while. Something of the old situation has to die. Often we see there has to be a new start with new energies. He called the Japanese lantern the "*church.*" This is the type that is displayed at the temples. This still has to do with the question of religion.

In the next session he had a dream:

> *I was sitting in the point of an upside-down pyramid. Stones fall all above.*

The last tray had the form of a pyramid, but it was not clear cut. It was rounded. Let's think about the pyramid. It is a tomb for the kings. It symbolizes the Self. The triangles come together in a square at the bottom. The body that is brought meets with the *Ba*, the spirit needed for the spiritual journey. So in the dream he is actually sitting in the Self.

Regarding the falling stones, Jung often described things falling from heaven as beneficial and spiritual. So sitting in the seat of the Self, this pyramid is like a baptism, a strengthening of the Self. Now he is in the Self. So this is his manifestation of the Self. This is very like Jung's childhood image of God defecating.

Through sandplay we can really come to these experiences. This is the main goal to achieve with sandplay, but let's not forget that this is just a beginning. It is the manifestation of the Self which leads to a new development. If we stop at this moment, we can be sure that this manifestation can be thwarted from the outside. It is not strong enough yet. It is an experience which gives us the possibility to develop a new side of the personality. Many children are very lively when they experience this and the parents may not want to take the child to the therapist any more. We tell them this is like new grass that comes up in the Spring. If we walk on it we trample it down. We must carefully tend to it.

Trumpets announce the arrival of the king. Something significant is about to take place. When you work with children listen to what they say. Do not ask them for anything. It all comes out. To ask them would destroy this inner growth.

## Tray 6
## Boy Age 12

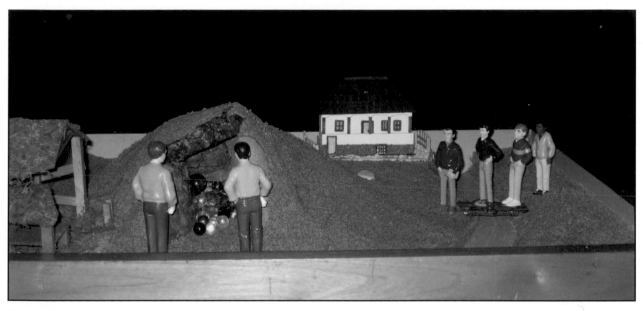

**Tray 6a**
**Boy Age 12**

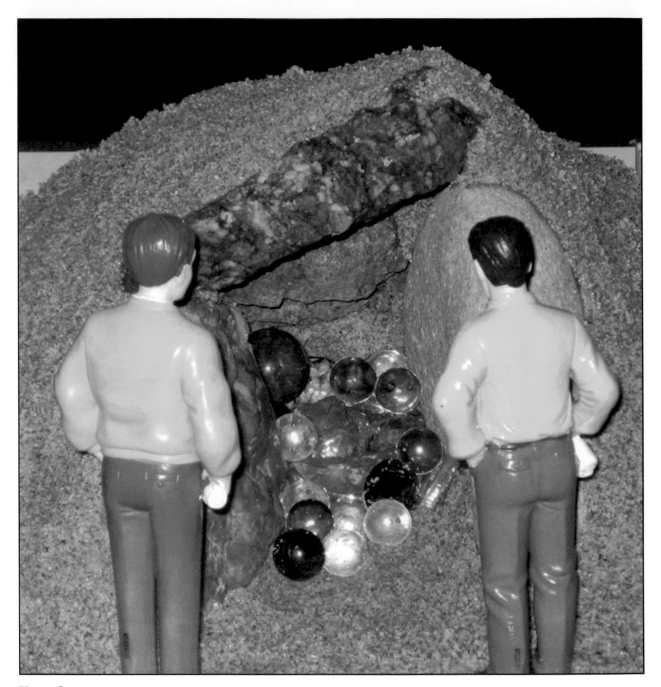

**Tray 6b**
**Boy Age 12**

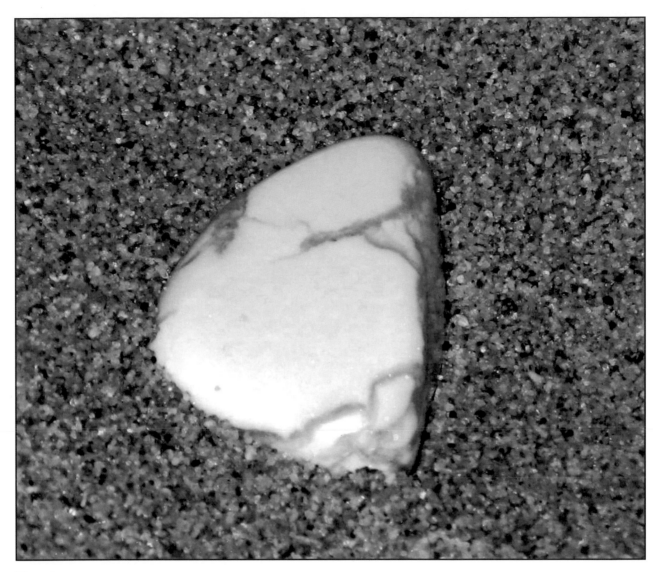

**Tray 6c**
**Boy Age 12**

*All of this belongs to a man. Many people come who want the jewels.*

Here we see the cave again, now made of solid stones. This is a very safe place in him. At the beginning this was a church. Now we have men instead of Smurfs. He invites the other people to come. He wants to share. When you are full of good things, you want the others to come and share. He shows here how the numinous experience needs to be shared.

Four men come across the bridge. This is completeness, wholeness. This is the totality which shares with the quintessence of the manifestation of the Self. Now this becomes available to him. These values that he has within himself are becoming available and he can share them.

We have seen that what is shown in the tray can be seen in the child's life within six to eight weeks. With adults it takes much longer.

The white stone refers to the Bible, where it is said you have a stone on which your name is written before you are born. This means that you belong to God. He may now feel that he actually belongs. Before he did not because he was not baptized.

The bridge is useful because he can walk from one side to the other. In the beginning there were big bridges, but guards prevented people from crossing. This bridge really looks like it belongs in the landscape.

The cave is very strong here. There is something very strong inside of himself.

**Tray 7**
**Boy Age 12**

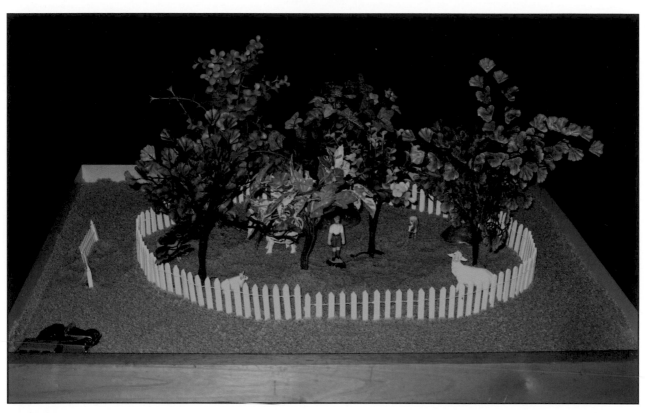

**Tray 7a**
**Boy Age 12**

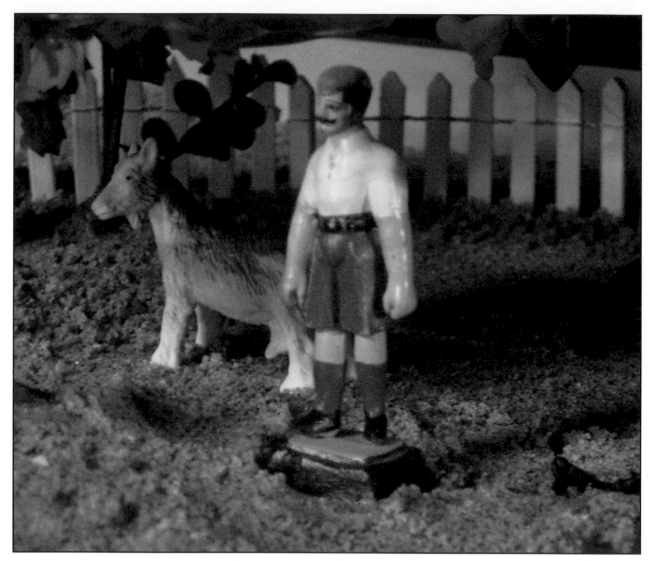

**Tray 7b**
**Boy Age 12**

*This is an oasis in the desert. Each year a new man comes and brings a new tree. There are very few people who know where this oasis is. One man lives here always.*

This is himself.

*The trees grew so fast that they had to cut them down. There was so much nourishment from underneath, that the men began bringing the animals. The opening is closed because there are six new trees that have just been planted and they should not be disturbed.*

He begins to protect himself.

> *One has brought an apple tree. There are twenty-two kinds of trees here. Water has to be fetched*
> *from underneath, especially when there is a war. They love to come here.*

This is in a desert, but here is a place where things grow and thrive. Although he feels he lives a dry, isolated life, here is an oasis.

Why does he bring mostly males here? When the ego is thwarted and is not in contact with the Self, the children have difficulty developing their own personality. It seems that this stands for a personality in the world, the masculine is his foremost development.

There is a female goat, which gives milk. It has a nourishing quality. There is so much nourishment here. After the Self is manifest, the first level of development is an animal, instinctive level. Here he brings the plants, animals and human beings.

Water comes from underneath, the unconscious. The unconscious feeds this situation, whereas before he was cut off from the unconscious.

If you live under a devouring mother, this is a negative feminine quality. From the manifestation of the Self you develop a better feminine quality yourself, so you are no longer eaten by the devouring mother. He showed this in the aunts that are disapproving of his developing the feeling quality of the feminine. He shows this in a softer way now.

Parents who take drugs have not had the manifestation of the Self. What they are looking for in the drugs is the spiritual quality. The drug problem is due to the lack of the spiritual quality in the world. We give our value to money instead of the spirit. In New York I was shocked when I was able to look down on the roof of a church. I found that so many insurance companies made the big buildings. I thought that our insurance used to be the church. Now it is the money. I lost everything in the war in Holland. When I came home I decided not to have any insurance, because I am the only one who things depend on.

## Participant Questions

*What do you think about having children testify in court cases?*

The worst thing to do is to have the child testify about their parents' drug problems. We need to work with them from within. We tend to give too much emphasis on the outside things, the courts and the system. Let us give the child a healing through his own work.

*How do you handle child sexual abuse?*

If the child admitted active molest, I would work with the child. Tell him that the father must not be in a very happy place, and work with the child. I am certain that the abuse would stop at a point. (*Editor's Note: This response greatly disturbed the group, as it conflicted with contemporary training in sexual abuse treatment and with regional reporting laws.*)

Sexual abuse is because there is no real feminine quality in the world any more. All the emphasis is on sex. Sex is not even lived the way it could be. It could be the most beautiful thing, but it can also be very destructive. Unless the man begins to appreciate a woman, nothing will change. But he cannot appreciate her if she wants to be like a man. It is really hard for us to even see what it means to be a woman. Women have been victims since the 13th century.

**Tray 8**
**Boy Age 12**

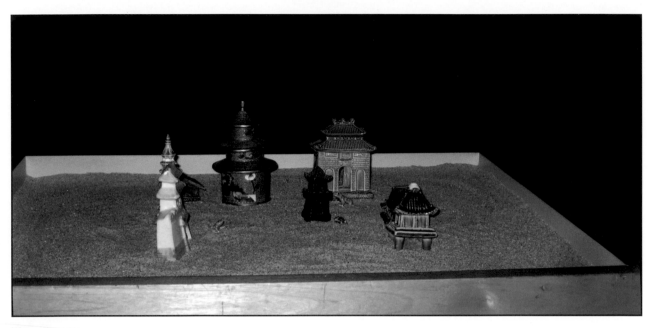

**Tray 8a**
**Boy Age 12**

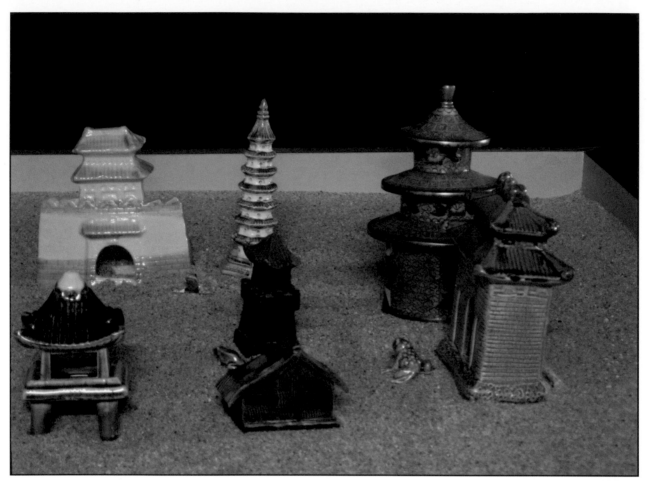

**Tray 8b**
**Boy Age 12**

*This is a city on the bottom of the sea.*

Frogs are the transformation to the masculine. The frogs become the prince. From the very depths he begins to develop his instinctual masculine quality.

This is a square city. Four is feminine and the square is feminine. Out of this comes the masculine quality. The feminine usually comes first, as the first contact is with the mother. Feeding through the breast provides a unity, a security with the mother. Neumann talked about this. We see the mother-child unity during the first year of life. The masculine always evolved out of the feminine in the old myths.

**Tray 9**
**Boy Age 12**

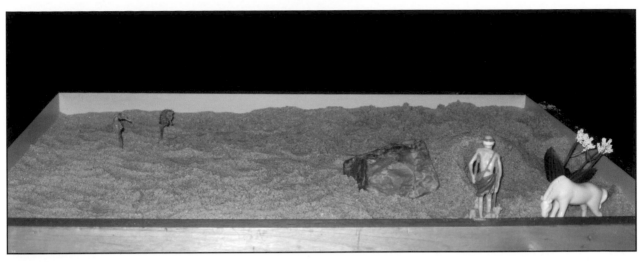

**Tray 9a**
**Boy Age 12**

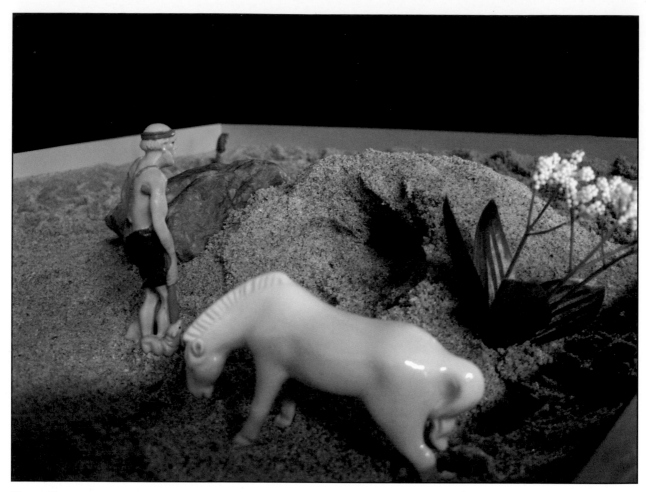

**Tray 9b**
**Boy Age 12**

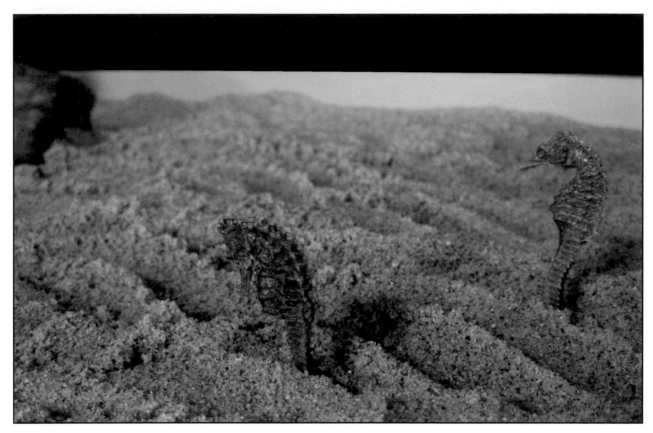

**Tray 9c**
**Boy Age 12**

*The poor man dreams that at the border of the sea where the white flower is blooming, there is his happiness.*

He talks about the poor man. He does not need the jewels; he has the jewels. This is his inner quality. But he needs the white flower and white horse – the numinous quality.

The two seahorses – the female brings the eggs to the tail of the male. He nurtures them for twelve days, then he gives birth. Two seahorses mean that he needs to become conscious of his own masculine nurturance.

After this he said:

*I will not come to see you anymore!*

He knew within that he was finished, even though his outer life had not changed yet. I always accept what the child says.

I always meet with the parents before meeting with the child. I never show the slides to the parents. But one time I had to show the slides to one family, because I would not have been able to continue with the child unless I had some information. I showed the parents and explained what was happening in a simple way. I went to Jung, who said that I showed the unconscious of the child to the unconscious of the parents. So, if we show the parents the pictures, we must first ask the child. Also, you must show it in a way that they do not feel guilty.

**End**
**Boy Age 12**

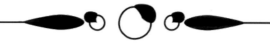

# Girl Age 16

## *Isolated with Psychosomatic Symptoms*

This is the case of the sister of the boy from the last case. She was sixteen and a half years old. She felt isolated and was new to school in Switzerland. She was in a clinic for psychosomatic illnesses for an ulcer in the duodenum and was referred to me. I saw her before I worked with her brother.

She was unhappy in school and was not thought to be intelligent enough to go to the gymnasium. (High school) I knew nothing more than this about her when she came to see me. I tried to talk to her, but she could not speak to me. Because she could not talk, I thought she might like to play in the sand. During the first hour I usually explain things, and do not ask them if they would like to play in the sand. But I thought this girl might like to put her hands in the sand because she would not talk.

## Tray 1
## Girl Age 16

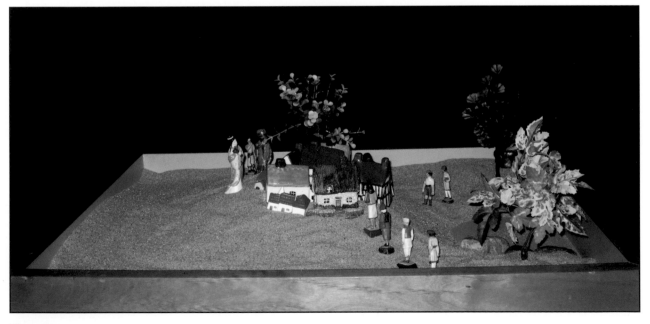

**Tray 1a**
**Girl Age 16**

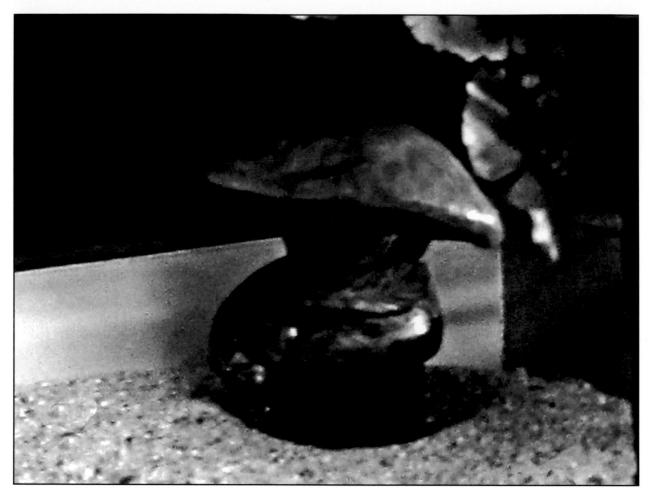

**Tray 1b**
**Girl Age 16**

People cannot walk in this city. All of the people are outside. All are from the Far East, East Indian and Japanese.

As a first impression, it is empty on the left. It feels lonely even though there are people. If this is a body, it is all constricted in the lower center. (Houses)

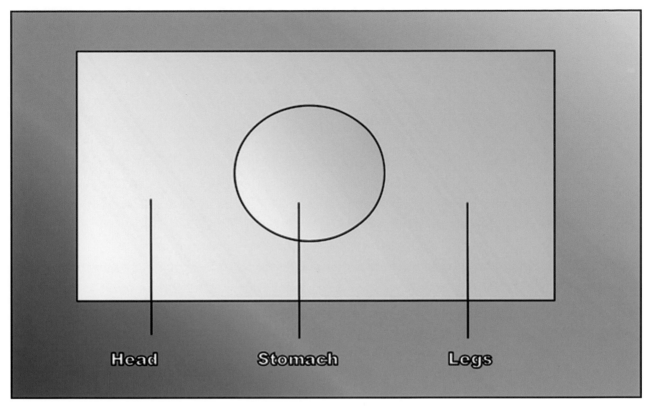

**Looking at the Tray as a Body**
**Girl Age 16**

All of the figures fall inward. There is no interaction. They are detached.

All of the people are foreigners. When people use figures from a different culture, we have to see how far away from the client's culture they live. Here we have India. This is half way to the Far East. They are in the unconscious, but not in the very deep unconscious. The Tanokami would be much farther away, so that would be something much deeper in the unconscious. Here it is not the conscious mind working, but she is already on a deeper level. When you see first images you can see this from where they work and by the figures they choose. People who choose figures from the Far East tend to go very directly to the deep unconscious level.

You can see that she is not conscious, that she lives in a different world. We can see why she would have difficulty concentrating at school, and why she would have difficulty making contact.

The village is right where the elevation in the sand is. This looks like it is in the tummy. There must be quite a strain in the tummy. I thought that there must be something that made her frustrated inside, but what was it? Maybe we can see the cause of this from the tray. All men and only one woman. We can conclude from this that there is a lot of masculine pressure. Maybe she lives under the influences of the rational education. Her daily life may be ruled by this. Some feminine quality is lacking, because there is only one woman.

The lake may be a resource. The swans start out ugly and become beautiful. They represent the union of the masculine and the feminine on an instinctual level. So here we can see that there may be some hope of bringing the two sides together from a deeper level. This could be an answer to the overpowering masculine side. The swan is a beautiful animal. It is very proud.

Tanokami is the guardian of the rice field and is said to live in the mountain. When the rice seed is put into the ground, he comes down to the rice paddy and remains there until harvest. He protects the growth and development of the fruit. When it is harvested he returns to the mountain. He is always shown with this huge hat. In the front we see him as a male, but from the back we see him as feminine. From the Far East, this is a very deep level of the unconscious. Deep within herself she has the capacity for this guardian and the union of the opposites. The meeting of the opposites is an experience of the wholeness of the psyche.

With sand pictures we cannot say that this is the masculine or the feminine side, the conscious or the unconscious side, because the sand pictures come from a much deeper level. We cannot say this is the consciousness and this is the unconscious. When we work from a deeper level, we work from a deeper transference. I do not think we can talk about this like that. Professor Kawai made a distinction between a grosser transference and one that is on a deeper level. Maybe when you work on the grosser level, maybe you can talk like this. However these are three-dimensional pictures and you cannot do this.

The center is much fuller than the surroundings. It could be that at this moment she is just more concentrated on this difficulty. What is around is not taken into account right now.

**Tray 2**
**Girl Age 16**

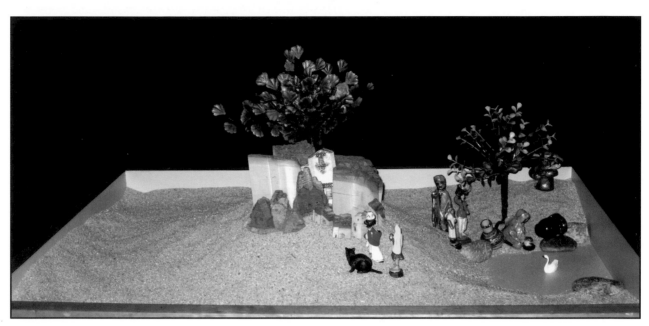

**Tray 2a**
**Girl Age 16**

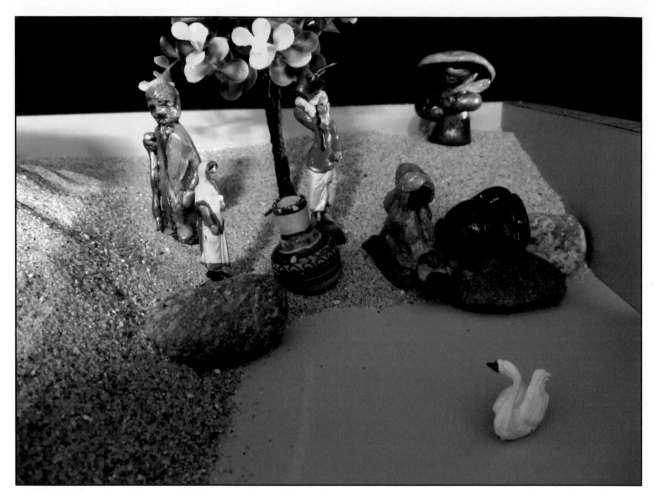

**Tray 2b**
**Girl Age 16**

This tray is very like the first, but most of the men disappeared and there are more women doing washing and going for water. The village is a little more open, but is still crowded. Things are opening to the feminine. I would think that she is more concentrated on the feminine aspect as there is much more feminine presence now. They collect water. This indicates that to develop the feminine is the answer. Because they are washing, they are active. These are all feminine qualities, because this is how Indian women really live. This is the answer to the overpowering masculine from the first image. The first tray shows us what brought her to this point. If we see this as the body, the duodenum is where this is concentrated. This shows us that she is only working from the duodenum. Perhaps before, she was working too much in the upper part of the body. But now she has a chance to work in a much deeper level. What we have here is actually the answer to the overpowering stagnation of the masculine. Here the feminine becomes active. Often at the beginning of analysis we have dreams of washing, cleansing. This means to clean the unconscious of all that makes it dirty, ugly or difficult. Here it is displayed with these figures.

The Tanokami is here. Maybe she looks for a guardian.

The black cat is the feminine. It is very independent. This is the dark side of the feminine, and here it is next to the village.

The Indian women are a feminine quality that is lying dormant within her.

Stones can carry the image of the Self. It is solid to hold on to. St. Peter is called "*the rock*." At the shore of a lake, there are often stones. This is a true image of a natural landscape.

This tray is more lively. There is an opening in to the village, a possibility of going in and out. The women lead toward the water. They are really in connection with the water, whereas the men walked away from it before. The water is becoming more important. It can signify the unconscious contents. The water has a strong transformative quality. It can be a psychic transformation of the inner contents, like a baptism to give the child the possibility to be of a Christian belief. Maybe water will begin to relieve her physical problems.

She is still completely withdrawn at this time.

This is still a constricted village. It is really tense. Something that forbids movement, or running through. It is still empty all around. This makes us think that this is the main problem.

**Tray 3**
**Girl Age 16**

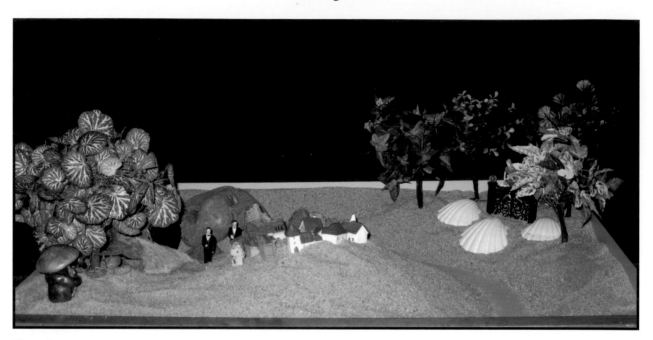

**Tray 3a**
**Girl Age 16**

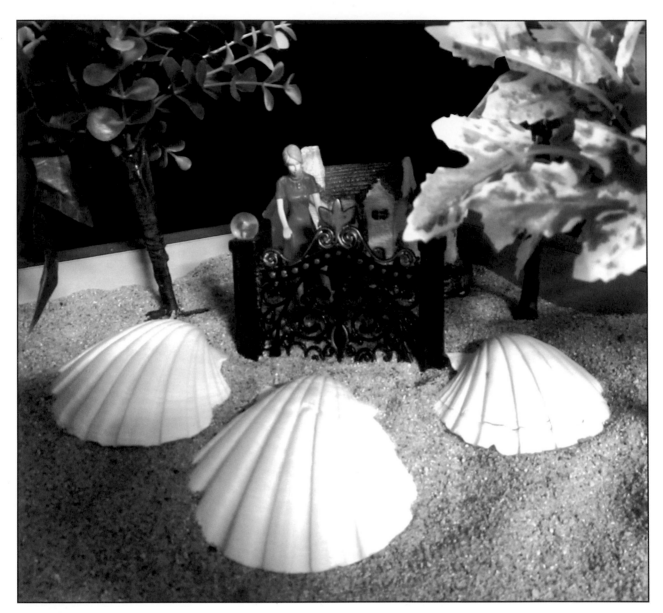

**Tray 3b**
**Girl Age 16**

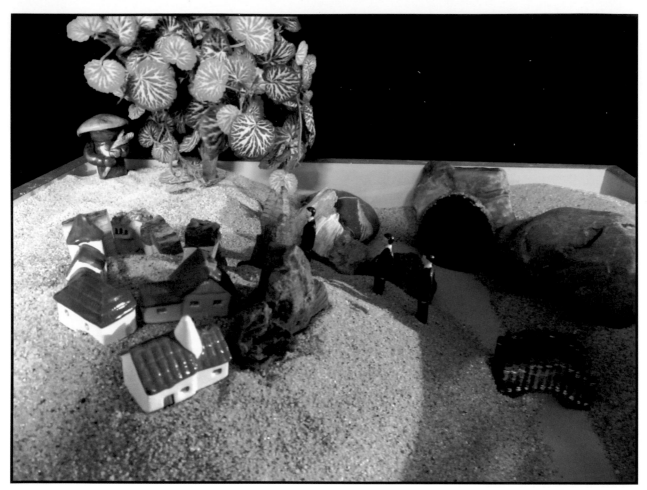

**Tray 3c**
**Girl Age 16**

She has no way to get to the village. Now the water becomes a river and begins to run. She tells us that she is in the picture, but that she cannot as yet go to the village. She is near a house. This is more modern than the houses in the more primitive village.

Because it is centered and empty around, we see that this is on another level of the unconscious. Now the tray is fuller. It looks more like a scene from daily life. I take her house more to mean her home. Maybe she tells us something about her home situation. Maybe she is kept back, not allowed to go out. This is more of an extension of the explanation of her problem. She is very near to this house. Maybe she does not dare to go out. Maybe she is not allowed to go out. Maybe something prevents the gate from opening to prevent her connection with the outside world. She tells us that there is no possibility to go from the inner to the outer.

The shells are in the way. Usually these are a wonderful symbol of the feminine. Why do they prevent her, block her way here? Maybe it is the mother. Here they are closed. (Turned upside down) There is no opening to the feminine yet. Maybe the mother has not been able to show her the path. Later I learned that she was nearly seventeen years old and still was not able to go outside of the house after school. I did not know this until later, but could tell this from the picture.

There is a round-shaped tree here. It is more like a fruit tree, more feminine in character. Here we can say that from the vegetative level, something is growing on the feminine side.

At the same time, she is kept back and not open. But on the other side something is growing. There are four trees, which indicate wholeness. Something holds back her development, and something is beginning to grow. At the same time the water begins to run. This is a big difference from that stagnant pool before.

Tanokami is still here. This is a guardian that watches something grow. Tanokami and the house are on a diagonal. The diagonal is very important for development. What we can see in the diagonal usually indicates that development is taking place. This gives us a clue about the development. The center is still the same here, but the picture tends toward the development of the feminine. In the center is the situation she wants to be in, but the seed is put with the feminine. (The shells and trees) The diagonal with the Tanokami indicates that she needs the protection for this growth and development.

The rocks are very large now. She is getting a hold on the protection that she needs.

## Participant Question

*Is the Tanokami a transference symbol?*

I do not like to see myself in the pictures, but it could be taken this way.

**Tray 4**
**Girl Age 16**

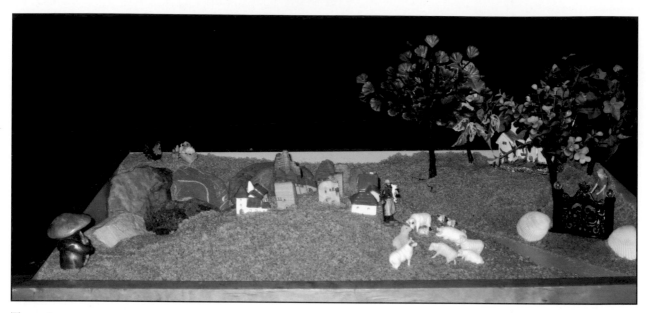

**Tray 4a**
**Girl Age 16**

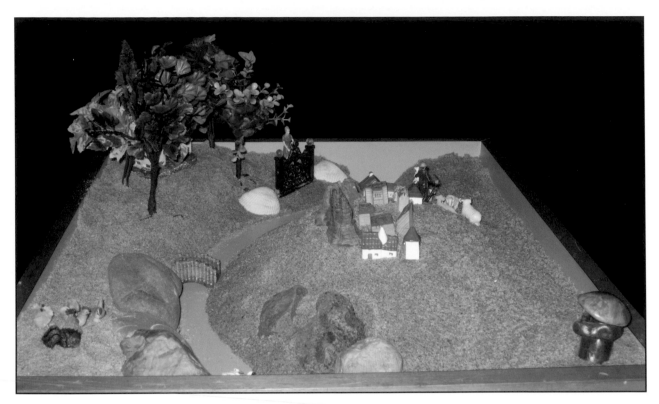

**Tray 4b**
**Girl Age 16**

Now the sand is wet. There is a masculine tree (pointed pine) here with the feminine trees. This is a growing integration of the masculine and feminine on the vegetative level. In the Tarot, number five is the Hierophant, where masculine and feminine are integrated. (Four feminine trees and one masculine)

What is different is that there is another tree, the girl is closer to the gate and the path to the bridge is more open. In the village there is now only the shepherd and the sheep. The swan is not alone, but there are ducks. Also there are chickens.

Christ is the shepherd who looks after the human beings. We are moving in the development of the feminine. The shepherd and the sheep inhabit the village now. Here I began to wonder if this had to do with the Christian belief, if this is a religious question. Here we now have a completely different masculine activity. Here it is the protector, the guardian. This shows that a more divine, or spiritual quality is coming up. Now she has a more open path to it. This tray feels so much fuller, but she is still not talking.

**There are various movements in the tray:**

- The pine tree points upward
- The girl moves forward
- Other animals are now with the swan and the chickens
- There is an opening in the village
- The shepherd and the sheep are the main figures in the village

There seems to be something with the Christianity, but at this time I did not know this. I only had these images to follow. It may be that the shepherd, which is the guardian in the Christian tradition, becomes more important to her.

The sheep are sacrifice, the Christ. They are animals that are always in a group. The first will be the guide and the others will follow. In Greek there is the word *próbaton*, πρόβατον, which means "*the go-ahead animal.*" They all move together. Because we see a group of lambs, we may see a going ahead.

The Tanokami is always present for protection and guidance. Now there is a shepherd for protection, too. She makes things clearer, because she shows what the problem is. (The Christianity)

Chickens have to do with eggs and fertility. They are on the same side as the girl. Maybe they belong to her. Because they are opposite the Tanokami, I thought that we might have to look for the meaning of the chicken from another culture. In Japan, out of the chicken grows a chrysanthemum. In the Shinto temple areas, there are many chickens. In Shintoism, the chicken is considered the most humble animal. To reach the highest level of spirituality, you have to be humble. This reminds us not to think about spirituality, but to come from the ground with it. The chicken is the divine quality that arises out of the humble attitude. There is something being prepared here that has a very different quality.

## Tray 5
## Girl Age 16

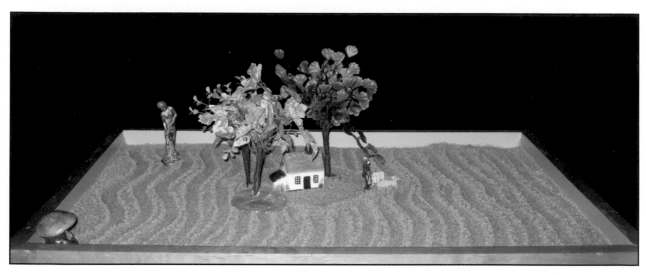

**Tray 5a**
**Girl Age 16**

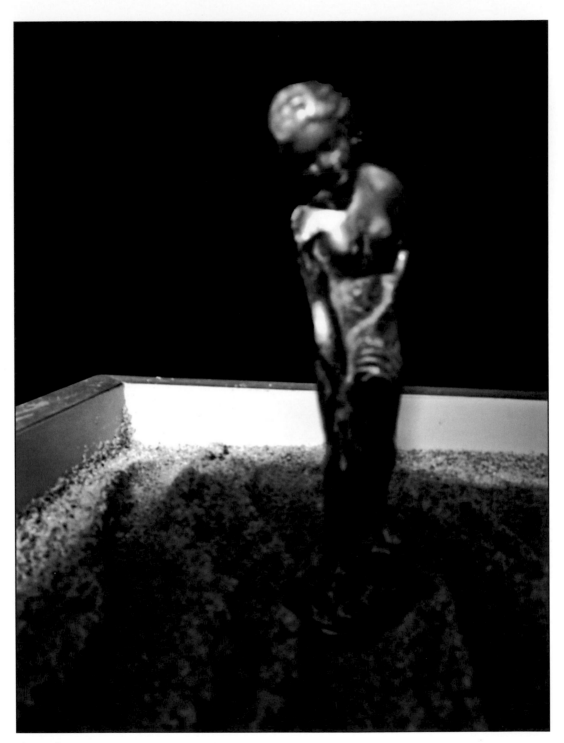

**Tray 5b**
**Girl Age 16**

This is where the shepherd lives. We can see that we are moving toward a religious realm. The shepherd is the main figure here, who lives in the desert where the wind blows and where there is great silence.

The diamond shape in the center is very basic, very clear. It becomes a symbol of the Self. There are two sheep, representing the conflict that needs to be made conscious. Here there is an atmosphere that is created by this image. The wind is a metaphor for God, the spirit.

She calls this the "*goddess of art.*" This may be representative of combining the masculine and the feminine. The goddess is feminine. The shepherd is Christ. Tanokami has always been standing in the corner. This is an androgynous figure, both masculine and feminine, and she always put him in last.

The artist is the one who interprets the divine. Here she comes to a central question of the human being, the divine quality with the union of the opposites. She moves to bring this together. She never talked, but always showed the issue. She was overpowered by the masculine. Then she made some movement. Now there is some concentration on the divine level. Remember her brother's trays? They were very similar. In his last tray, he ran his fingers through the sand. Two trays before that he had an oasis.

Two weeks later she completely changed. She talked and said she had a dream with a fiery wheel that demonstrated a great light.

**Tray 6**
**Girl Age 16**

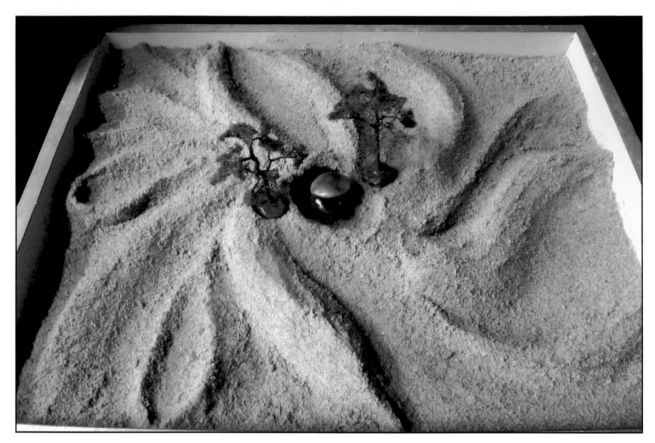

**Tray 6**
**Girl Age 16**

The phallus of the Tanokami is now in the feminine cave. It is like a lingam and yoni, which displays a tremendous light. The movement has come to the center.

The Japanese trees mean "*eternity*" in Japan. This is the eternal question of the human being to come to the center where this inner security, this relationship with the divine is shown. This is in all of us, the basic question. The closer we move to the center the more secure and happy we are. See the beauty, the strength in this tray? This is the Self tray. Now the ego can develop from this point. Now this is the vulnerable time. We have to see that it is preserved so that the new ego structure can be built up.

The fiery wheel is the manifestation of the Self. It is a union of opposites and it displays pure light. We often see illumination with the manifestation of the Self. It is then that the original Self is touched. The original Self has always been in us, and will ever be. It is the guide of development and the guide of the ego. The ego is always in contact with, and is guided by, the Self. It is this that guides the ego's development.

What is different after the manifestation of the Self? See, we always have an ego. The ego has to know that it is but a part of the Self. In the West we tend to give the ego the main power. It can be very strong as long as it is in connection with the Self. It can be strong in a negative way when it is not guided by the Self. This would lead to overpowering righteous situations. A negative animus, for example, is always "right." The negative animus always has the last word. We would like to transform those negative working energies into constructive positive ones so they will be helpful, instead of disturbing, or thwarting us. There is tremendous change and transformation after the Self has been constellated. Because the Self contains everything, the good and the bad, it is full. We see new energy available at that moment. You will see children become more lively, more outgoing, instead of sad or depressive. It is a great mistake to end therapy at this time. We have to take care of the development that arises out of this experience.

In the case of this girl, she was suddenly able to talk and to discuss things. When the manifestation of the Self occurs, people sometimes want to keep it, to guard it. Let's see what she did afterwards.

## Lingam and Yoni

In Hinduism, the *lingam* is a phallic-shaped stone worshipped as a representation of the god, Shiva. It is revered as the manifestation of the masculine creative energy. It often sits on bowl-shaped stone, known as the *yoni*, which represents Shiva's consort, the goddess Shakti. Shakti is the feminine creative energy. Together the lingam and the yoni represent the coniunctio of masculine and feminine principles, the wholeness of creation.

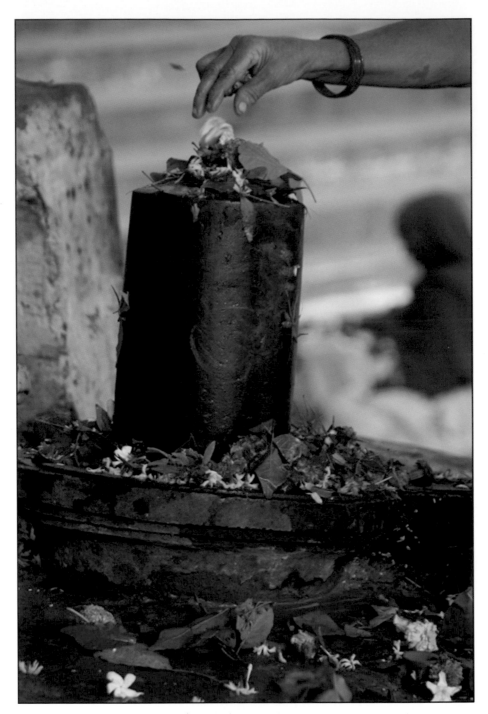

**Lingam and Yoni Worship – Varnasi**

**Tray 7**
**Girl Age 16**

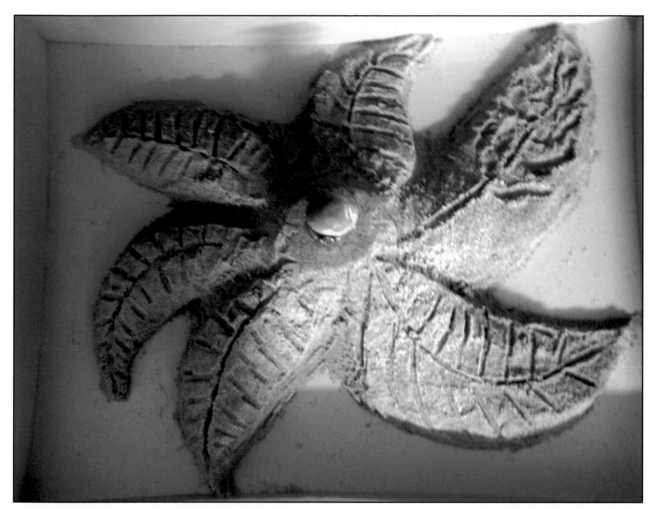

**Tray 7**
**Girl Age 16**

The flames have become leaves. Usually after the manifestation of the Self, the next step would be on an animal vegetative level. Here we have the leaves. This is still not conscious at all.

In Hinduism we hear about the kundalini energy. It is often shown as a snake coiled two and a half times around itself. It lies dormant in itself. It is not only life energy; it is feminine energy. When it rises up it reaches the animal vegetative level. When the kundalini reaches this level, it is said that the individual can heal himself. The healing capacity from within begins to take place. With sandplay, chakras begin to open. Here a lower chakra (on the animal-vegetative level) begins to be activated. The manifestation of the Self can be seen many times during a lifetime, but what is important is what a person does with this development.

I had two people who came when they were kids and again when they were in their twenties.

The Hindu tradition does not talk so much about the feminine qualities. But in Tibetan Buddhism they talk about the creative (feminine) energies.

The Dionysian experience is a moment of breakthrough.

A real mandala has specific measurements and it expresses a divine moment. It is a union of opposites, of god and the goddess. (Describing a Tibetan Buddhist mandala) It is a square with four entrance doors, south, north, east and west. Then in the meditation, you go beyond your daily life thoughts. Then you come to the clouds. The monks do this meditation to overcome their fears of death. They will often meditate on grave yards for days and nights. Then they come to the universe. I showed the Dali Lama some of these sandplay pictures and he said it was an experience of the Buddha nature. I showed Gopi Krishna some of these pictures and he said they were a kundalini experience.

**Tray 8**
**Girl Age 16**

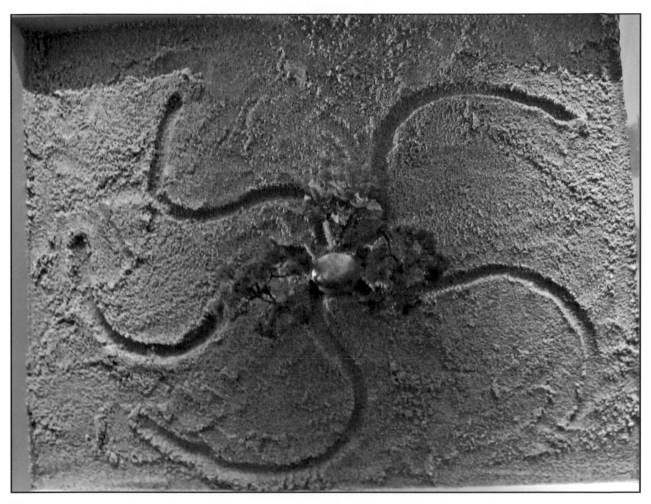

**Tray 8**
**Girl Age 16**

If this really moves counter-clockwise, it could mean that she really keeps it inside.

With the experience of the Self we have a psychosomatic healing. I have seen depressive people begin to breathe much more regularly after the manifestation of the Self. There are many psychosomatic healings in this work. I am sure there is a complete interweaving of the body and the mind. Even doing sandplay is an experience of the body and the mind.

**Tray 9**
**Girl Age 16**

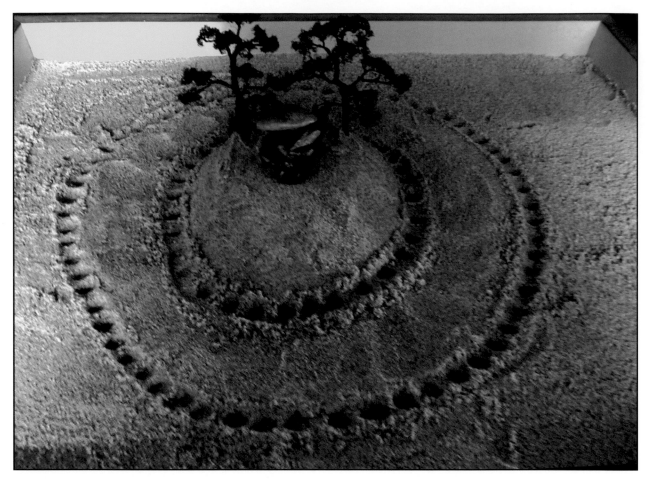

**Tray 9**
**Girl Age 16**

I feel that this was her last effort to try to hold on to this experience of the Self. I asked her what Tanokami was doing here. She said, *"He is the one who brings the sheep when there is enough food."* He is the shepherd.

The doctor called and there were no more ulcers. Her experience was so strong that she cleared herself of a very difficult situation. There was a new wind blowing through her with new energies. She showed what was negative already. What is here is a breakthrough toward something new.

**Tray 10**
**Girl Age 16**

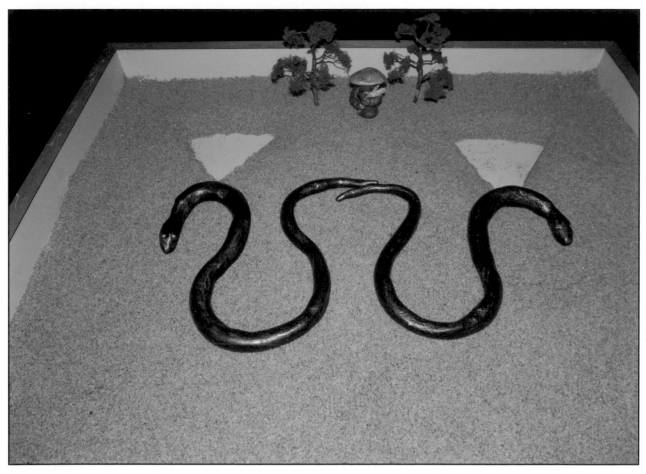

**Tray 10a**
**Girl Age 16**

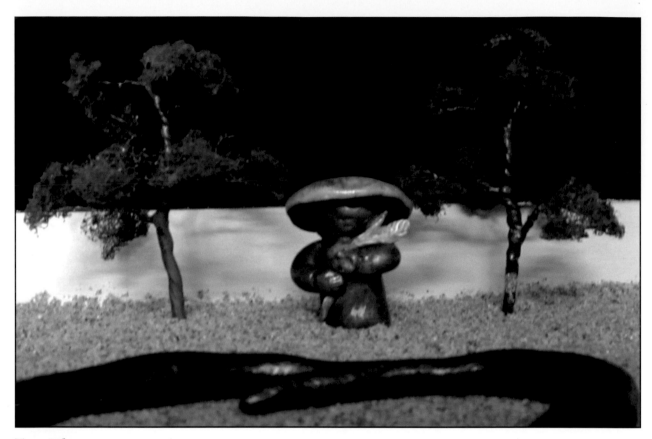

**Tray 10b**
**Girl Age 16**

The picture looks like two dancing women and a uterus and fallopian tubes. Here the real feminine qualities are displayed. Recall the first picture which was occupied by men. This is an opening. One feels like breathing here.

There are two triangles here that point down. This is seen as feminine, especially in Hinduism. The Tanokami oversees this.

At this time she said she was really kept back by her family. She was not able to go out after school, meet with friends, etc. I suggested that we might find a different school which was farther from home, so she would have more freedom. She said her mother would never allow such a thing. I asked her if she thought it would be a good thing for me to talk to the mother.

I talked to the mother and told her that her daughter was kept back and would have no chances of developing if she was kept in this school. Later the mother agreed.

With this tray she began to live. This opens up her possibilities. There is much more water in this tray. The prior trays had more of a fire quality.

I think we can talk about the opening of the feminine creative energies here, through the experience of the total personality. This was what was lacking in her.

The word *kadoma* is Tibetan for kundalini. (The feminine energy, literally "the sky dancer." Mind in its total aspect as Self.)

The figure in her tray is an ancient Japanese symbol for medicine. Later this girl became a doctor. Also without the triangles, this is the shape of the clasp used in Tibet. When you go to the temple, you get a little Buddha which you hang from the center of the piece. Jung always said that you can only bring your patient as far as you have grown yourself. This is a never-ending process.

## Tray 11
## Girl Age 16

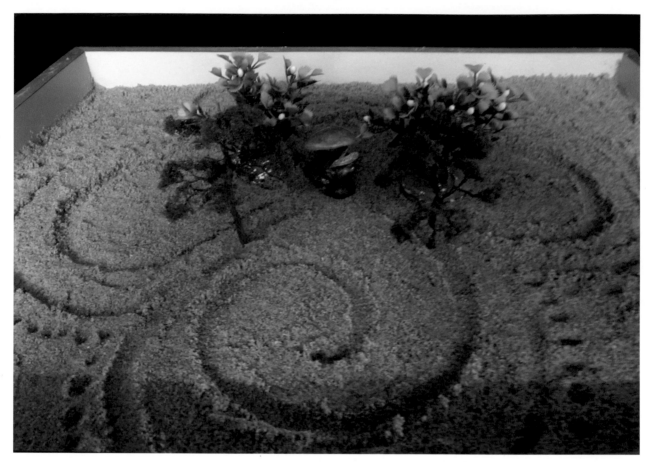

**Tray 11**
**Girl Age 16**

I feel there was a certain necessity because of her illness. This is why you see so much movement from tray to tray. When it goes fast and intensely, as in this case, it shows that there is a tremendous inner necessity for healing. This happens also when people come from America, as we work three times per week. We have to remember that it does not show on the outside immediately.

In this case I see that there is an indication for development given by birth. When we reach the deeper levels, it shows. When the person is able to experience this deeply, we have a bigger chance that they will be able to realize it in the outer world.

This tray even looks like the movement in the digestive track. It could be also that she was beginning to digest this experience. I also saw a treble clef in the tray. I asked her if she played an instrument. She did not but said she wanted to play a stringed instrument. Later I found her a teacher.

She has finger pokes on the left, and finger tracings on the right. The pokes look like a honey comb, a little hole to plant seeds in. Tanokami is still here. The tracings look like a terraced rice paddy - like furrows. This is like an imprint in her that the seed may grow. Again, it is very strong. I was amazed at the force of these trays. This was why I wanted to talk about it; otherwise it could become another tension for her.

(Regarding the shapes in the tray) The intersecting figure eights are twice the sign of infinity. They are the four directions of the world.

You can see how interconnected these pictures are. There was always a development taking place out of the last one. When we see a picture we can look to see where that development is taking place from the last tray. Here we can see the clover leaf shapes in the prior trays. The violin scroll design.

**Tray 12**
**Girl Age 16**

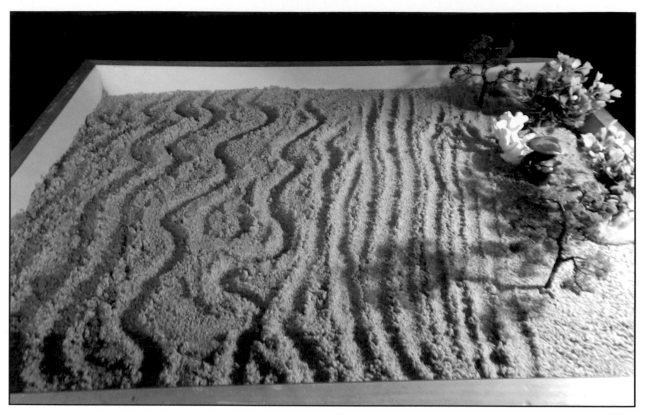

**Tray 12a**
**Girl Age 16**

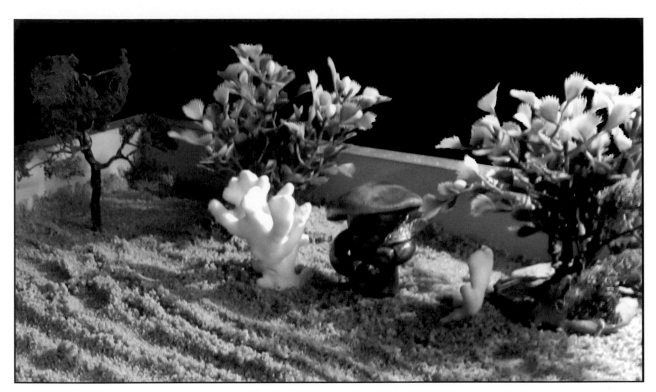

**Tray 12b**
**Girl Age 16**

Tanokami has moved to the side now. It seems that he is preparing to leave. (Now that the seeds have been planted)

The white coral and jewels have a feminine quality. The jewels are from the depths. He (Tanokami) takes the jewels from the depths. He has achieved something. Maybe it is a gift that has been given to him for having been with her. Maybe he wants to take something from the deep sea up to his mountains.

The waves in the sand may be the subtle division between the two, like a border. Maybe it is a labyrinth that she knows her way around in. You can see some movement. (In the tracings in the sand) There is some movement in her.

At this time it was decided with the parents that she would change schools. We chose a private school that had kids from other nationalities.

**Tray 13**
**Girl Age 16**

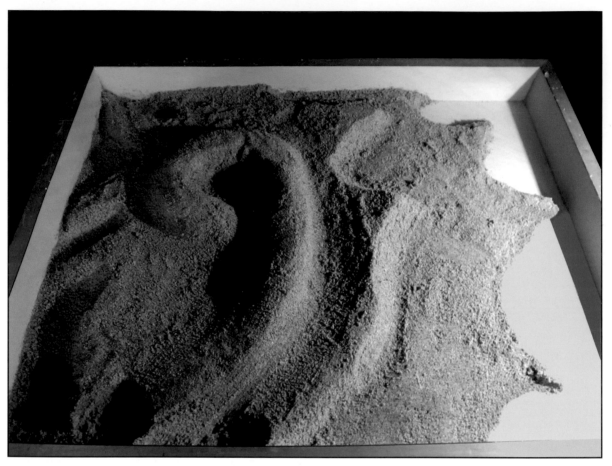

**Tray 13**
**Girl Age 16**

There is a very strong intellectual capacity shown here, as well as a strong feminine and sun-star.

Tanokami is gone. She has integrated it. She is beginning to be very strong. She can apply these energies that she has. She began to be better at school and began to play an instrument. Now she could go to school for the whole day. I had to give her a chance to live with these energies she was discovering. (By suggesting she change schools) The family began to shift. This was my family therapy.

I only see one child in a family at a time, as they would get jealous. I saw the youngest brother. In the first tray he made a bass clef then covered it with wood, plants and animals. Only after you uncovered all this stuff could you see the clef.

**Tray 14**
**Final Tray**
**Girl Age 16**

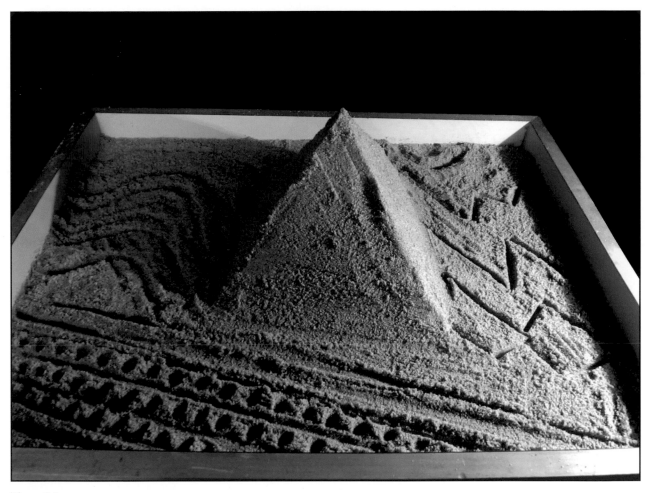

**Tray 14**
**Final Tray**
**Girl Age 16**

There is a place in the pyramid which receives the first shine of the sun in the morning. It is in the chamber where they have put the mummy. They say these walls are beautifully smoothed and polished, like a mirror.

The scarab's journey is from sunset to sunrise. It is a night journey.

It looks like rays of the sun and furrows. Like her brother, she said she was done and would not come any more. Once you have achieved such a process, you can bring it into the outer life. You must give people the chances to live it in their daily life. This is the therapeutic purpose. It can easily disappear if it is not put into action.

Do not go through the slides too soon. (With a client) The gap between the conscious and the unconscious will be too great and it may have a bad effect.

**End**
**Girl Age 16**

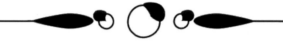

# Woman Age 46

## *Depressed with Negative Animus*

This case is an American woman of forty-six years. She felt that a man would save her. She was very self-critical and had a negative animus. She was depressed. She was the middle child in a family. The mother was stylish and sexually liberated, and her father was a *puer*. They had divorced.

Her only childhood memory was a rough treatment by a nurse. One month after her son was born, her husband was killed. She returned to her grandmother's home where the grandmother dominated. She remarried when the son was five. She did not love him and divorced after seven years. She re-married three years later, but her depression increased, and they divorced. She thought she was crazy and sent her son to me for therapy. After two or three sessions he asked if I did not think he was normal. But he said, "*You should see my mother.*"

She cried because I was three minutes late for the first session in the States. After that she took her last dollars and came to Switzerland. I saw her three sessions per week, because she needed the contact. At the beginning she could not touch the sand. She was afraid of the material. She said that she had several dreams after I first worked with her. She had studied to be a teacher, but said she could not take in any more information. She would not be able to earn a living unless she passed her exams.

Here is her first dream:

> I am in a wood paneled room. There is a red haired man with a beard sitting on a chair with his face averted. There is a smaller room adjoining, separated by a wooden banister. A couple comes in. They are Mexican. They give me a large, heavily carved wood ring. Two keys are hanging on it. At the organ in this alcove, the organist tries to play, but my cousin is fiddling with the keys. I ask the man for something and he tells me it is in the cupboard above. I get on the chair and look into the cupboard and cannot find anything because it was only dark.

The Mexican couple can be the instincts. They bring her the ring, wholeness and the keys to unlock the mystery. The Mexican couple has to do with something lower in the body, something she is unaware of.

Something becomes available in her unconscious, not in her daily life. In daily life she asks men for the answers, but finds the cupboard dark.

The averted man is available, but in a negative way. This is the emptiness. A positive animus is not available. It is empty and dark. She still takes directions from the man.

She stands on a chair looking up for the solution. She is looking in her head. Her animus is occupied completely with learning. She could not do any more. No wonder the man in the dream looks so unhappy.

The wreath, or ring indicates that she can probably bring things all together and make it complete. It is wooden and hand carved. This has to do with the hand instead of the mind. This is a very good sign.

The two keys are the creative, feeling side she is missing in her daily life. She needs the feminine. She must develop a feminine, maybe a creative side, because this wreath is handmade. It is artistically carved. But she had no access to this at this time in her daily life.

## Drawing – Dream II

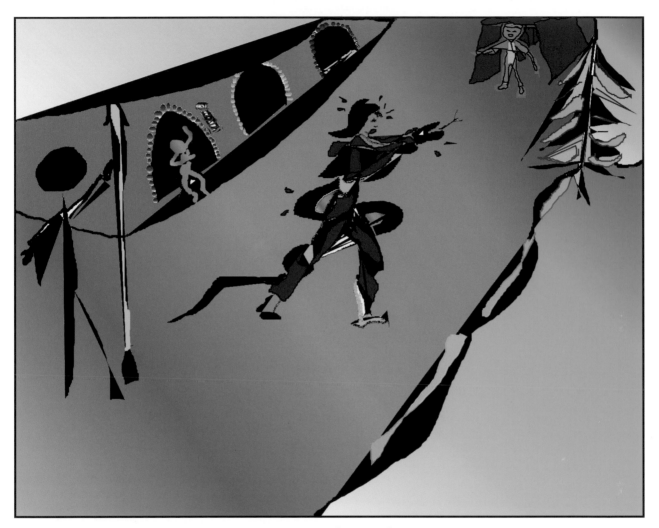

**Woman Battling Snake**

*I am in a little Mexican town. On the right side is a park. A huge snake comes at me and we begin to fight. It is the worst fight I ever had because I know I must not give in. I got hold of his neck and managed to hold him away from me, but we are both getting very exhausted. We almost give up. He bites me a little on the shoulder, but now it is going to be okay because there is a tent not far away. This unknown man will know how to clean the wound. As I go up the street, the barber comes out of his shop and is amazed. No one has survived the snake before.*

She is in a Mexican city. She went into the unconscious. In the park, the plaza, she encounters a huge black snake. This is the dark, shadow part. She has to hold it and control it. The shadow wants to overcome her and be stronger. This is why all is dark in the cupboard. This is a very strong, negative force in here. She has to try to hold it a little away from her. The snake bites her. She gets a little venom to build an immunity.

The unknown man is the masculine side that she does not know yet. She has to develop this and side with this masculine quality. She fights with the negative side that is known to her. But there is another masculine side that is at a distance that she may contact after the fight.

The trees are masculine growth, a positive animus in the future.

Dreams often show the path to take. We have to deal with the things that are told in the dreams. If we do not pay attention they will appear repeatedly until we find a way to pay attention. In sandplay when the therapist does not recognize what is going on in the sandplay, you will see repeated trays. The unconscious mutual understanding does not take place.

I feel that the understanding of the sandplay takes place in a synchronistic way. There is a mutual understanding on a deep unconscious level. When this takes place the next step of the development can take place. With the mutual, unconscious understanding, it is not necessary to speak about it. The therapist has to be aware of it. There is a play between the two persons. Even if you do not understand completely what is going on, you have to get a feeling of the experience yourself. This is how it goes. Then this is often enough.

She begins to fight, to be active. Her feet are now more on the ground. She has more color. She is in Mexico. So now she is in the unconscious and her unconscious had more color. She is on a deeper level.

With dreams of being in a foreign country, see how far this is from our own country. Look at the cultural differences. See what is there to heal the conscious situation in the unconscious details.

The barber is traditionally a healer. He represents the path to the Self. He brings order to the hair, often seen as thoughts, opinions. When they put it in order, they put the thoughts in order. This is why they are healers. They used to draw the poisons out of the body.

Mexico is on a sub-conscious level, because it is not completely down south yet. The culture is very different from America. It represents the earth of America. It was there that the Aztecs and Indian people lived. It can therefore be on a deeper level because it has to do with the earth quality. If

Americans get in touch with the people that have lived before in their own country, they will get a lot of knowledge for their own development. It is different when people live in Europe on their own earth. They are more in touch. This is different and more difficult for Americans than for people who come from Europe. They live in America on the surface. You need to get in touch with something deeper. So Mexico represents the earth for Americans. Therefore it is quite deep. To value the Native American cultures will give us a sense of what it means to live on this earth.

The woman had cut herself off from this deeper side. She had always looked for a man who earned a lot of money, one that was conquering this earth. After we cut ourselves off like this, then we begin to search.

## Drawing – Dream III

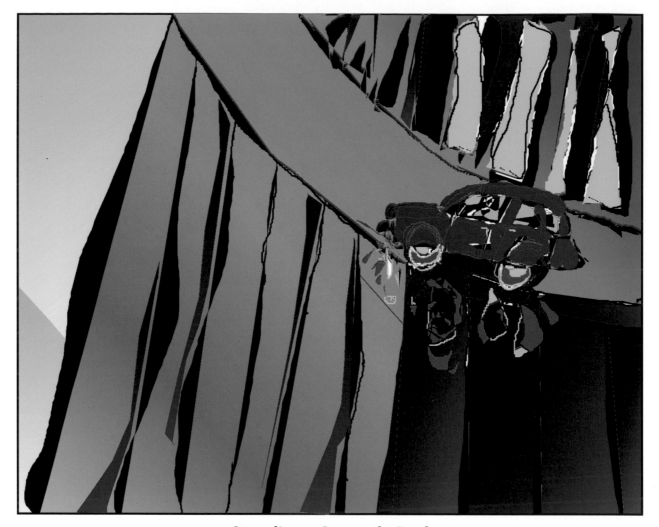

**Struggling to Stay on the Road**

*Just before falling asleep, I was driving over mountains where I drive whenever I leave town. I was in a struggle for my life. There is a force pulling the car over the cliff. I resolved to struggle and not go over the cliff. It was so frightening I was so glad I did not have to drive that road before I left for Switzerland.*

She was probably afraid to come to Switzerland. When we undergo such a big thing we do stop and wonder if we are doing the right thing. I think she was near suicide. This force that takes her toward the cliff is likely her suicidal tendency. She is at the edge of her being at times. She was in the driver's seat. She can handle it herself.

If we think of negative things, this may influence the client. We have to be the strong force that keeps them alive and keeps them going. If I do not leave a door open, they have nowhere to go. She is going down, but is controlling her descent. She is ready to go into deeper levels in herself.

## Drawing – Dream IV

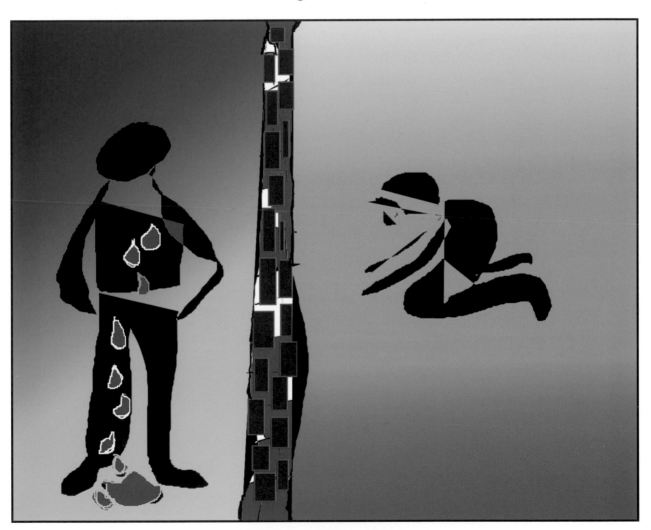

**I Cannot Stand It Anymore**

She drew herself as a motionless sad woman. On the other side there is a man.

> *I am trying to show how I feel inside. The woman is sunk down with her forehead. No energy. The man is dressed properly, but the demands he makes on me are impossible. I cannot exist without my blood flowing. I cannot pretend any more. I can't stand this anymore, so put a brick wall between them.* (Man is bleeding from his heart)

She was a very attractive woman. I felt that she would be spoken to in the hotel. That is why I wanted to see her so many times a week – so nothing would interfere with the therapy.

The man is bleeding from his heart, because his real masculine side is really hurt. There is such a big difference between the outside and the inside of this woman. From the outside she looked so beautiful and put together. So many people hide their pain.

After this she made her first sand picture.

**Tray 1**
**Woman Age 46**

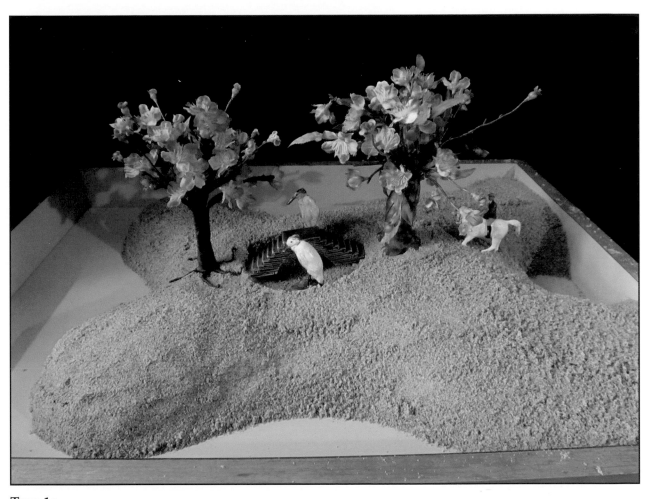

**Tray 1a**
**Woman Age 46**

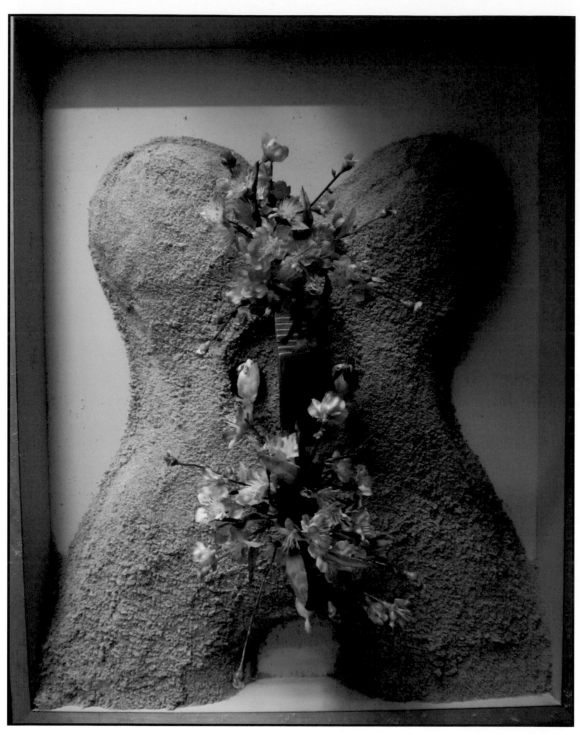

**Tray 1b**
**Woman Age 46**

The man comes from underneath and the head is gone. Women who have been very rational will often do headless bodies in the sand. I had a female medical doctor who did a headless body and was ashamed of it and wanted to cover it up. She was so far away from her own body. I was shocked.

She is in the middle of her tummy - before she looked for something in the upper cupboard. Now she is in her body and makes a bridge between the upper and the lower. This is her rescue, to make a union of the lower and the upper part. Therefore there are so many Japanese flowering plum trees. They are the first to bloom after the winter snow. There are given the symbol of perseverance. This is a beginning of a flowering in the middle of her body.

A man comes on a white horse. This is the divine quality. This will be a completely different animus quality. It does not come from her head but comes from a deeper place in herself.

The heron symbolizes long life and spirit. It is an indication for a completely different development in herself from the middle of the body.

The whole body floats in the water. It feels calm. You can see how she waited several sessions before she began with the sandplay. We have to wait until they are ready. You have to be inwardly ready to work with the sand.

## Tray 2
## Woman Age 46

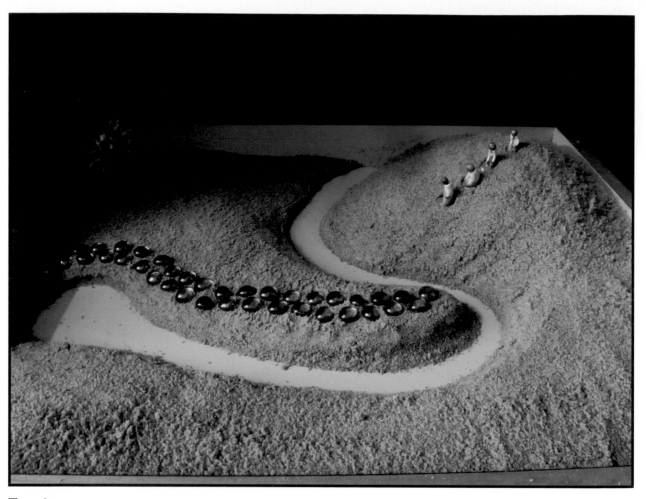

**Tray 2a**

**Woman Age 46**

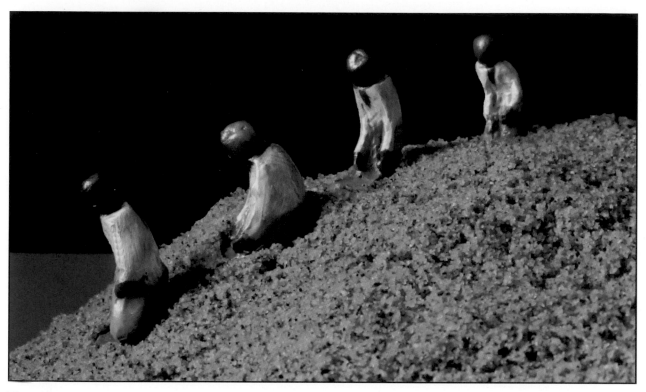

**Tray 2b**
**Woman Age 46**

*They are putting the seed into the ground for the rice field.*

The animus qualities step down from the hills to plant the seed in a lower part of herself. Rice seed is planted in water and earth. These are two specific elements that she works with here. When we talk about the five elements of our body, these are the two lowest. Earth is the lowest. Medically, organically this corresponds to defecating and urinating. Next is the water level, which has to do with the kidneys. We can see that she is moving toward the depths in herself. Often we see direct indications of the level from which they work. Earth and water have to do with working in the very deepest part of the unconscious.

## Elements of the Self
## From Buddhist Tradition

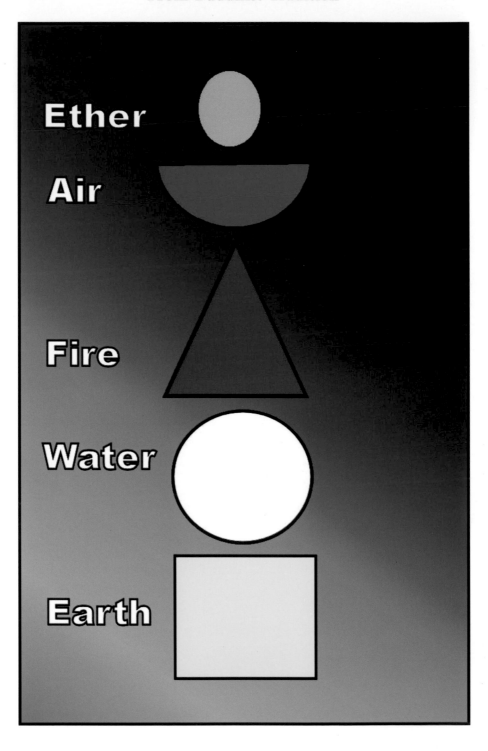

| Element | Color | Qualities |
|---------|-------|-----------|
| Ether | Blue | Space, Spirit - Sometimes flame-shaped |
| Air | Green | Talk, Noise, Lungs Breath - The mind in contact with the body |
| Fire | Red | Heart |
| Water | White | Kidney |
| Earth | Yellow | Bowel & Urine |

This shows the functioning of the body elements and is also the structure of the five-story pagoda. In the Far East, the body and mind are seen together. In the West, we have separated ourselves from the body.

This lady is at the beginning, with the mind. She had forgotten the body. Now she puts the seed in to the two lowest elements of the body.

It is very interesting to see on which level the pictures are made. For example, someone wants a lot of water, or earth. Sometimes they want to make a lot of fires. Ayurvedic and Chinese medicine are based on the five elements. There is good health when the five are in harmony. When one is overpowering, there is imbalance. For example, too much fire and water is hysterical. Acupuncture can help bring the elements into harmony.

You can use meditation practices that go from the bottom to the top. Visualize a glowing thread which arises from the bottom. *"Au..."* (Chanting) *"Oooohhhhh..."*

It comes up and becomes hotter, until it reaches the head where it becomes the *"...Hummmmm."* (Chanting)

Then the glowing thread melts the *"mmmm"* and they go together down to the heart.

Sandplay deals with the water and the earth, which we have neglected for so long. You can only become spiritual through the body. We have nothing of that in our churches. Sandplay may be a therapy which begins to get in contact with the elements of the body.

## *Participant Questions*

*What would you think about a client of mine who burned paper and liked watching the ashes rise in the air?*

The problem seems to be with fire and air. We can see on which level the difficulty is. The rage comes out because he does not have enough love. The element of fire can be healing, destructive or transforming. When the negative fire element is present you can transform it into a positive one in the therapy. Just as Mara became the enlightened one, energies can be completely transformed in the work with the sand.

*Will you please address the issue of clients who use a lot of water?*

People who use a lot of water can make it very hard to clean, but be sure to accept it fully. Then they will be able to stop that later. When they do stop observe what they are doing next. The free and protected space contains the permission to live through the problems, but with someone who gives the space and the limitations. If it goes too far, you must reduce it and keep it within the client's limits. Some people can go further than others. We must recognize how far we can go. Where is the danger? If the water becomes overwhelming and he never stops, there is a danger that he gets overcome by the unconscious. Look to see where the signs are that this will be reduced in the future.

I had a boy fill the tray up to the top with water. His father had killed himself by throwing himself under the train. The boy did not know how he did it. Believe it or not, he always put one train track in the tray then filled it with water! This became less and less. One day he did not put the rail, but the sand was soaked. Then he put in a little dog. This was such a good sign. The dog is the nearest instinct we can handle and guide.

We have to see what made the situation like this. Then we can see if the work is going in a good direction or not. You must always be hopeful. Do not think it should be good, but hopeful. When the clients say they are feeling hopeless, I will tell them that I will hold the hope for them until they can take it back for themselves.

*Could you please talk a little more about the element air?*

Air comes from people who like to talk a lot. Maybe they have been silent before. As in the previous cases, the girl did not talk for quite a while. Finally she talked.

*Can you tell us more about the element ether?*

Ether is displayed during the whole therapy. In a way it is the attitude we have for a feeling function, the free and protected space. We are the therapist with the good spirit for helping this person. Then the Self can bring the numinous qualities to the work. Then this goes with the person. Sometimes we see more spiritual figures in the sand.

I often think of my clients between the sessions. They are with me a lot. Then I have to cut it out, so I can leave an empty space to make room for something else. Between clients I always walk through the house to clear one client from the other. It is not good to just stay in the room and have a new client come in.

*How long should we make the sessions?*

I see clients for forty-five minutes. This gives fifteen minutes between to take photos and clean up the trays.

**Tray 3**
**Woman Age 46**

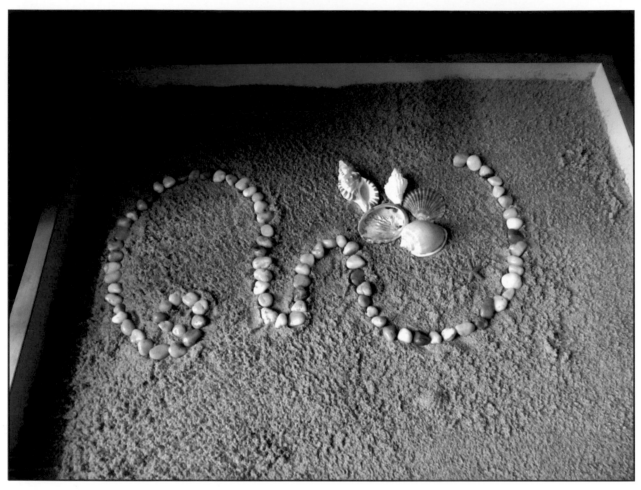

**Tray 3**
**Woman Age 46**

*This is the bottom of the sea.*

She is at the deepest part of herself. This is very revealing because I could see that at the bottom she has a feminine quality. In her deep unconscious, she is not deprived of the feminine.

The five shells correspond to the five elements. I felt that the total aspect of her was actually feminine, because we had the chance to go very deep.

The sea star is the totality - the five elements. Living here in the depths of the sea, in the depths of her unconscious, she is actually feminine. It is just in her education and her outer life she is being so masculine, rational. This one-sidedness thwarted the feminine from being integrated. This was where the depression comes from.

Depression comes when you depress qualities that would help you be more fulfilled. We have to find where these qualities that are suppressed are. So her femininity is really at the bottom.

The woman is born feminine. But we have to develop the masculine. Then they have to be in touch with each other. But if the culture emphasizes the masculine, we have to bring the feminine quality up to a higher level. This is our task. We have an enormous power in our hands. The feminine is not valued. If we do not fight for it like a man, that is difficult, too. I do sandplay in my home so people just think this sandplay may be okay just for children. (Not in a man's way, in a business office)

We are ourselves not so aware of what is lacking, because we live in this society. I only came to see what was lacking through the sandplay. The feminine is a lost quality. It is hidden; it is in the dark. The more we recognize where these qualities are, the more we will be able to penetrate and bring it to the surface to integrate it into the masculine, rational side. The rational side needs the nourishment of this feminine side.

### Drawing - Dream

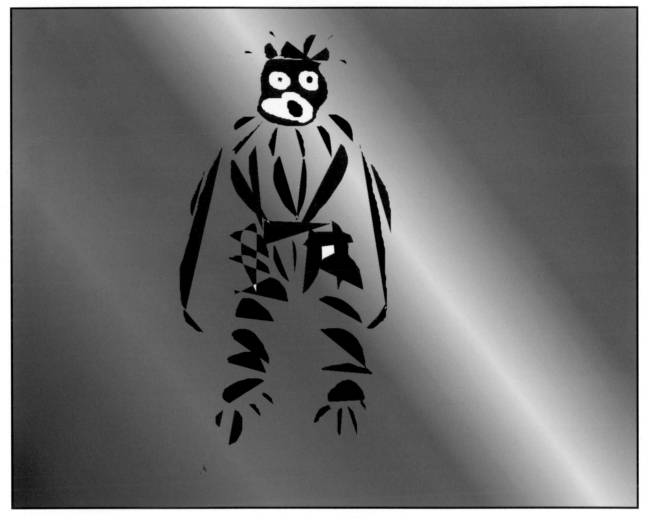

**Large Scary Monkey**

She did a drawing of an ape, or a monkey. She was very frightened, so I did not want to leave her in her fear. I had to tell her about the different qualities of the monkey. We can see that it is brown. It is dark like the earth, whereas the snake had been black. This is different from the monkey. The monkey can be playful, or it can attack. Because it was a huge figure here, I thought it was a very important thing that I wanted to show to her.

The story of the Monkey's *Journey to the West* describes the monkey king, born out of a stone egg in the mountains. It was a miraculous birth and he was destined to be a special animal. The monkey undertook the journey, because he wanted to become the Buddha. The book describes all of the adventures. It is the basis for the basic teachings of Buddhism. So it was an animal that wanted to become a spiritual being. It shows that it is only through the animal-vegetative, instinctual level we can develop a spiritual function.

Because she was so frightened, I told her about this. Think back to the white horse in the first tray. There was an indication of a spiritual force coming from underneath. This happened after she had shown her feminine quality at the base of her being. Then she calmed down.

## Drawing - Dream

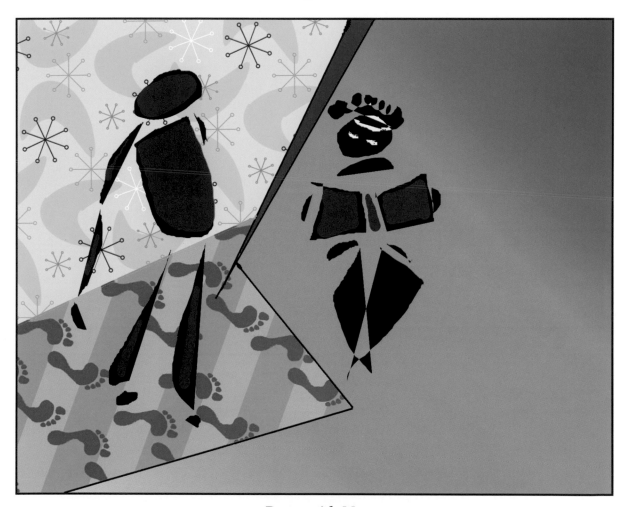

**Dance with Me**

*I was reading a book when a dark brown man comes to me and says, "Please come and dance with me."*

At this time she had calmed down, but it is not yet integrated. She is still studying in the dream. She dreams that someone comes to take her away.

## Drawing - Dream

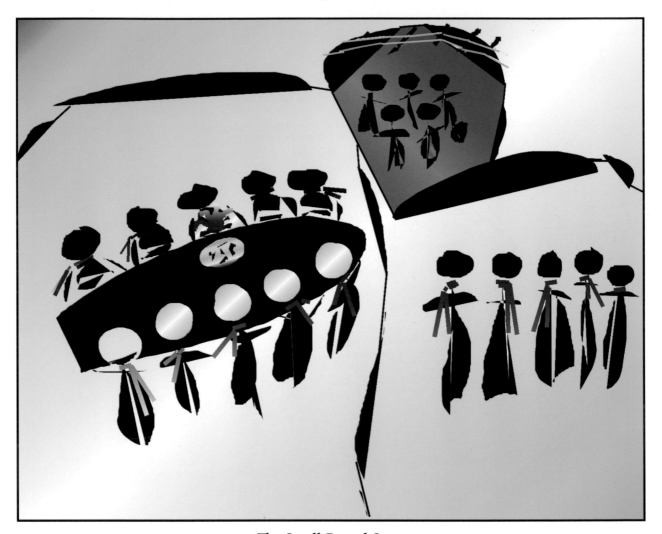

**The Small Round Stone**

*A small quarter inch black, circular stone had been found in the earth. This meant that a new religious leader must be chosen. A conference of all of the religious leaders was called. My godmother was there. An individual woman was there. All were in robes sitting at the tables when something fell into my lap and burst into flame.*

You see, this is the next element.

*I knew that this was a sign that I could lead. They could make me the leader of the boys' school.*

She knew that she could become a teacher.

*The boys were playing football in a tunnel under the railroad tracks. In the next room, all of the leaders had blue scarves around their necks. One made a sign to me, but I was content that someday they would acknowledge me.*

Do you see how the monkey had this religious quality? It came to her. I was also aware that she had no relationship to any religion, but when I saw the white horse coming from underneath, I knew she was in need of this. This is also why I explained the monkey to her. She did not acknowledge it immediately, but it came back to her.

Here the flame is tiny, not destructive. Maybe it is a healing, the beginning of a new development.

The black stone is like in the boy's tray before. They did not know each other. The archetypal level was activated here. So we have now the developmental stages. Development is archetypal. It is in all of us, if we are prepared to be developed. But we do not always have the chances to develop. In sandplay we have the chance to get in touch with the archetypes that lead to this development.

**Tray 4**
**Woman Age 46**

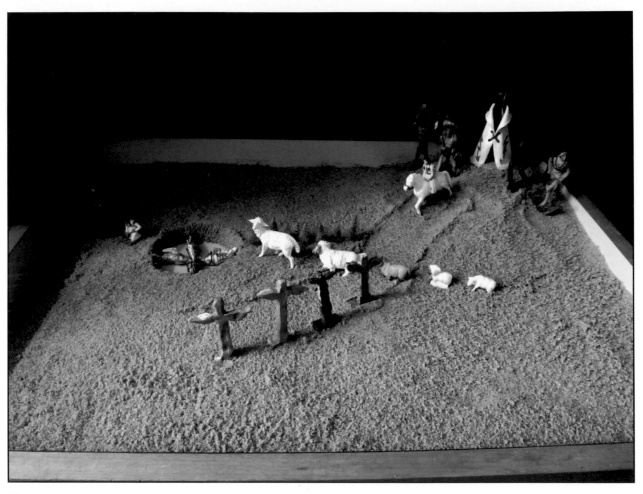

**Tray 4a**
**Woman Age 46**

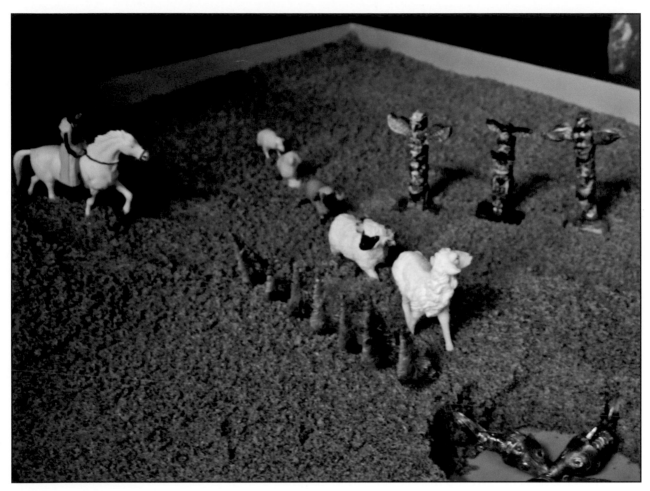

**Tray 4b**
**Woman Age 46**

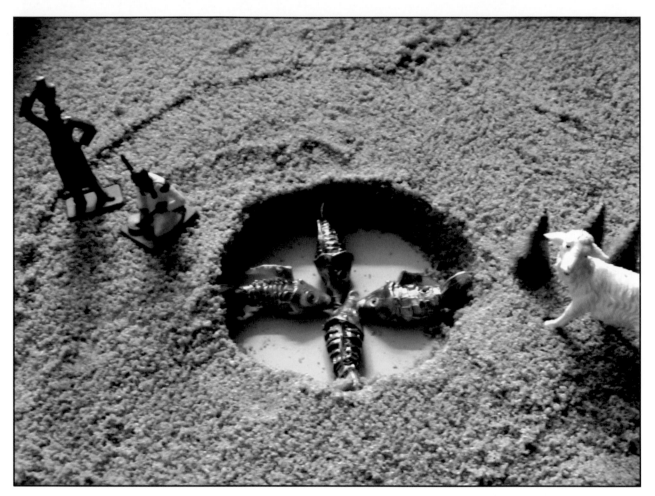

**Tray 4c**
**Woman Age 46**

She called the lake a closed crater. She did not know what was in the middle. She sees herself as an Indian woman who has to go on a journey. The woman carrying the water carries the unconscious, and the woman who is cooking carries the fire element. She leaves to find the feminine qualities, traveling along the four totem poles.

The totem pole is about the family belonging to the tribe. Indians belong so strongly to the tribe. As individuals, they are not so important.

She felt adopted into her family. Maybe now this belonging became quite important. After this she finds her individual qualities as a woman, carrying water and the fire. It does not mean that this is all the woman can do, but it is dealing with these lower elements and it is from there that she may find her totality in the crater, in the depths. This is a wonderful display of what she actually has to do. She longed for that. She had to leave the collective.

She crosses the line of sheep. This is the go-ahead animal. The quality of Christ, the sheep is sacrificial. Maybe this is her need for religion that she must discover, or come across. She has to sacrifice in the cross, in the sheep. What she has to sacrifice is this one-sided attitude.

After this tray with the Indian woman having to leave, she was especially tired. When you really work with the unconscious, the unconscious does the work and takes the whole burden. This is why some people get very tired after working with sandplay. She came to this crater which was a symbol of the Self. It was so deep down she felt that something profound was going to happen.

When she went home, she slept and had a waking vision of four huge snakes looking at her. She was not afraid because she felt she had a protected space.

## Drawing Vision

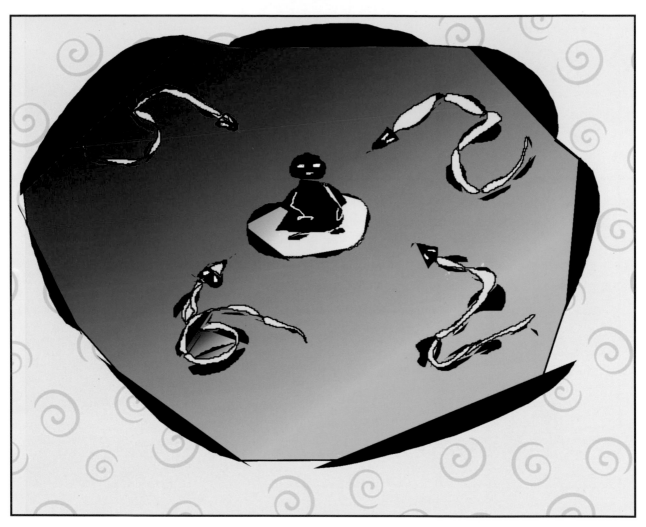

**Metanoia**

She is in the center in a protected circle. The snakes are now black and yellow - before they were just black. This means that these are beginning to change. She felt that something was changing. This is *metanoia*, transformation. It means to return to the beginning. This is why she was getting tired, because deep within her unconscious a change was taking place.

## Tray 5
## Woman Age 46

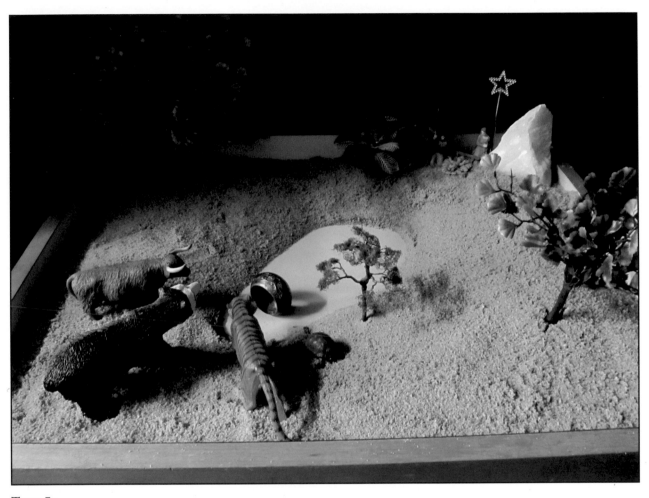

**Tray 5a**

**Woman Age 46**

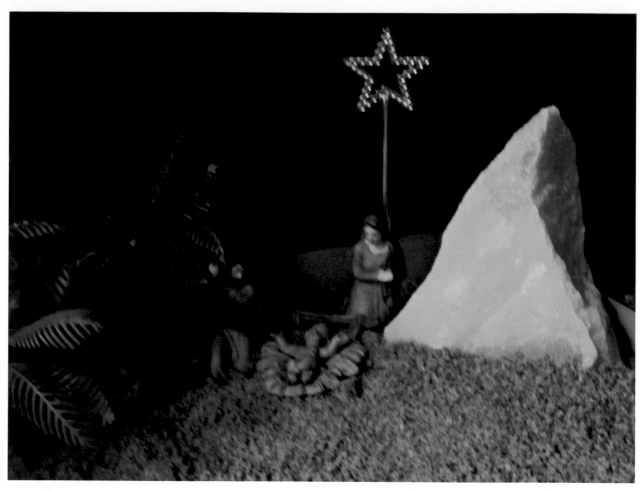

**Tray 5b**
**Woman Age 46**

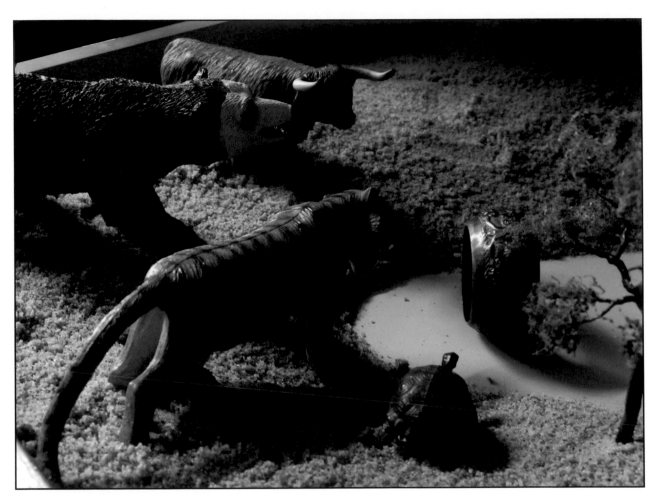

**Tray 5c**
**Woman Age 46**

She says this is the birth of Christ. All of the animals come to this ring to drink water. An instinctual force is coming alive. She is getting in contact with it now. Why is this happening at this moment? We should see this in the picture she makes. She experiences the divine child within herself. When the Self gets constellated there is always a numinous quality. This is the moment when our primordial numinous quality is displayed. This is a very deep experience and has a strong effect on people. I always ask in the last session what religious practice they come from. Is it the same as the ancestors, or has there been a change? Because when the Self gets constellated, it usually is accompanied by the original religion that they are from. It is the main instinct of the human being, according to Jung. Whether you practice religion or not you are still coming from this tradition. Even if it was only the ancestors that practiced it there will be symbols of that religion.

In the other case there was the fiery wheel and the Tanokami. She was baptized, so she chose a figure that represented a total aspect of the masculine and feminine. They can choose a figure or an expression that shows something different, but points to a totality. I am always overwhelmed when this happens. The people are overwhelmed, also. They search for a certain expression of their completeness. This is what the religious symbols are. This is the basis of our being. Jung said we were born with this. We yearn for this completeness. Through sandplay we can go so deep that the original Self gets constellated. This is the manifestation of the Self. This is the beginning of a new development, because the new ego grows out of this totality.

After this, the next step of development is the animal-vegetative. We can see here that it takes place in the woods, because they are showing the unconscious. On the other hand we can see the animals coming in, getting water. This is the basic nurture of life.

Overly rational people are usually cut off from the instincts. This is so common today.

## *Participant Questions*

*Is there a manifestation of the Self in all cases?*

It depends on whether a person has reached a totality or not. Those who have gone through that before, through life experience, or education, or whatever, will continue their development from another level.

*Does the manifestation of the Self happen several times?*

This is so. We can reach this level under new circumstances and have this experience at different levels. But usually people come to sandplay because they have had a deviation away from the Self. So they need to come back. This is a circular path that may repeat itself several times during this life. Jung compared life to a spiral. You come back to the same things but at a different level.

If a child is in therapy for one year, there will probably be just one manifestation of the Self. At the manifestation of the Self, children often ask for creative work. We do enameling. This is like an alchemical process of transformation. Then they have a jewel that they may want to give to their mother or father, whom they hated before. We do wood burning, also. They may want to play in the yard with balls, and so on.

You can see that they begin to be very constructive, whereas before they might have been destructive.

Sometimes you will see long, never-ending wars with children. When I think that this is going on too long and they really do not need to do it, but are doing it out of habit, I will make a correction. When it becomes more realistic than ordinary play, they may stop. In the sandplay I had one boy who kept fighting. I finally put caps under all of the soldiers. We ignited them and it looked like a real war when it was over. That was the end of his shooting.

*How do you feel about having guns and weapons for the children to play with? The most violent children I have seen are the ones who have not been allowed to have army toys at home.*

There is a phase of development that has to fight in order to get ahead. They must be given the chance to live this out. I tell them that it is better to fight when they are kids than when they are older. I give them the chances to do this in the protected space.

Neumann talked about the fighting phase, after the animal-vegetative. This is the phase where the dragon has to be fought. Girls do this differently. They want to ride horses and take care of the horses. With girls I felt that the phase is more of a feminine development, in that they not only want to ride the horse, but to take care of it. For the boys it is to fight and protect.

When we work with the sand, the process is to go from a conscious side and to enter deeper and deeper levels. This is why we will see the animal-vegetative level, but with a negative part. When they have reached the Self, they will come up again, but usually in a positive way. There is a transformation taking place from the manifestation of the Self, if we can live it with the client.

*Would normal, non-conflicted children show this in the sand, too?*

Normal children would likely just show their current situations that they are in, because they have manifested the Self earlier.

*Can we use sandplay to assess and diagnose children?*

Lowenfeld developed sand work to test children, the "*World Test.*" My special recognition was that I found this to be a process. You can use sandplay to get information about where the person is, but I do not think this is what we can best use sandplay for. I get an image from the last tray about where the client likely needs to go, but I do not just stay with this. I go on to see how the whole process evolves in the sand.

*Can we let our own children play in the sand? Or have an open sand tray for the children at school?*

This is fine if you do not look at it to see what is going on. In the beginning I said, "*No, no one can go in.*" I remember that Martin did amazing things in the sand. I feel pity that I did not take pictures of it. If they are free to express themselves it may be valuable. Martin did the arrival in heaven after death. If this is going on at school, I would advise them to have a much bigger box.

We cannot act as therapists for our own children. We are the same blood. Even Jung said to me, "I cannot deal with my children." I think we should never try. We cannot easily be objective and we can get the wrong view.

*What is a "normal" child?*

They are adjusted, but they may be adjusted to something that is not at all normal. Normal would be when you can always combine the two sides.

*What about doing research in sandplay?*

I would like to see that more people would be able to observe this path that is given by birth. If we touch this realm, we have more happy, satisfied people. This will bring people to a better life. So research that could look at sandplay in this respect will be most valuable.

*What do you think about taking notes during the sandplay session?*

It is best if you have your own experience of going into the depths and changing. From there you can feel the client's experience and observe them better. When we see what change can take place and we have undergone this ourselves, we participate in it.

*When we are introducing sandplay to the public, does it contaminate the process to show them cases?*

It does not matter if you show cases to the public, because they will always take it in their own way.

I once had a four year-old child with night terrors. She put a rabbit in the sand and played with it. I took her to the farm next door to look at the farmer's rabbits. She said she wanted, *"This one."* She cuddled it and loved it. She fed it. She came four times and each time she wanted to see the rabbit. After four times, the rabbit was gone. I asked her what she was seeing at night that was so scary. She said she was at the top of the stairs and saw two gods at the bottom. She said, *"They want me to come."* I did not know where to go with this.

She was at the time of the manifestation of the Self. She was bi-cultural, Japanese and American. These were the two gods. You see that the white rabbit has the same meaning in both the East and the West. It is the feminine side, which has access to the divine in both religions. This is why it would be so difficult to make research on this, because the child will take what is healing to them at the time.

## Tray 6
## Woman Age 46

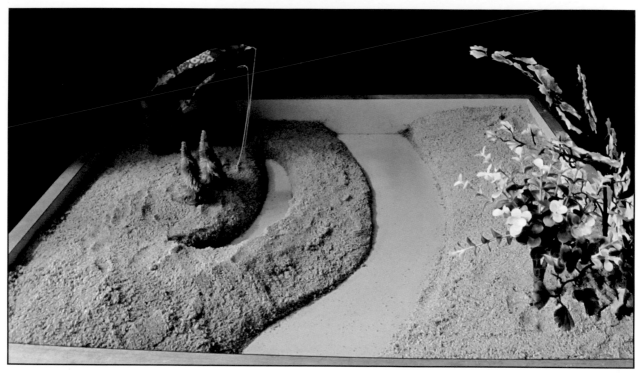

**Tray 6**
**Woman Age 46**

This is water and earth, the animal-vegetative level. It is an absolute beginning.

The Japanese flags with the carps come from the East. This is from deep within the person. The carp is the masculine in Japan. When a boy is born, they hang out a flag with the carp on it. When Western people go into the depths, they will choose Far Eastern symbols. In the East, the people will show Western symbols.

With the new element of the animal-vegetative level the new element of the masculine in the woman usually appears. This is a sign that she can develop a new kind of animus. Originally she had to battle a very dangerous snake. That became less dangerous and now we see a new element in a positive way.

This is the beginning of an ego development, which of course, comprises the masculine side. The masculine was there before but it was experienced in a negative way. In the woman the positive masculine means making judgments from a positive, feeling level. There is artistic possibility.

This flag is only used when the boy is born. Then on *Boys' Day*, all of these flags are hung outside the houses. On *Girls' Day*, there are alters with beautiful dolls on them. So this is why I think that we have to see this particular flag in this way.

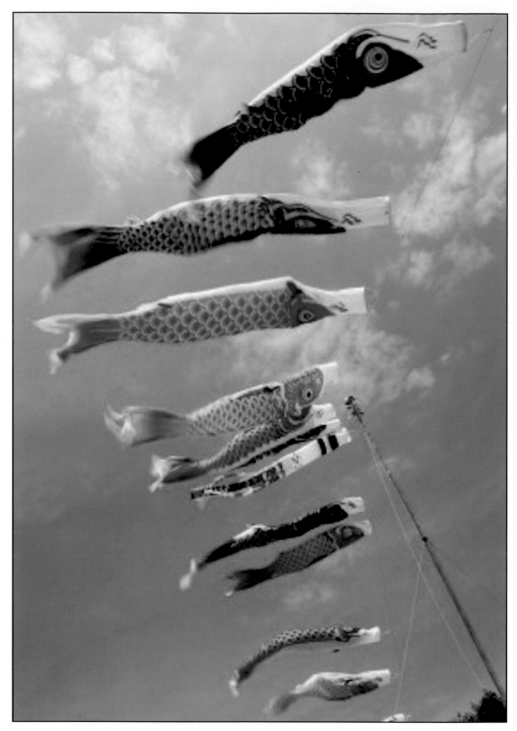

**Boy's Day Koi-Nobori Flags - Japan**
*Photo 123RF No. 6409161*

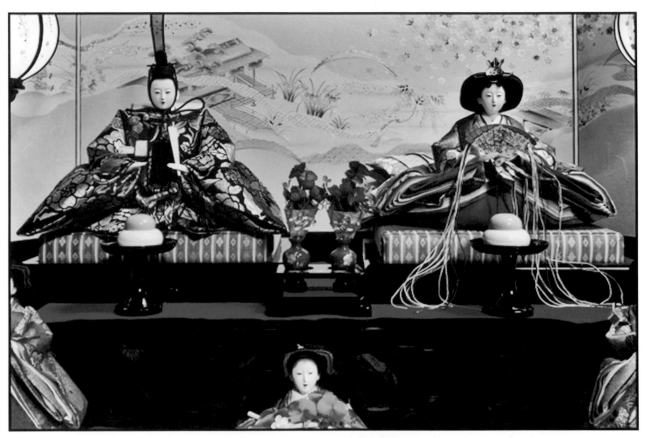

**Girls' Day *Hinamatsuri* Dolls**
*Photo 123RF No. 13982937*

---

### *Participant Question*

*Now that she has an ability to contain and protect the feminine does this mean she will be able to contain herself better and will not be going around looking for this in a man?*

She has to keep it in herself before she can make another contact. For example, it would have been too early for her to have taken those exams at this time.

Also, this looks like a new moon. So the feminine and the masculine are beginning. See in my book and compare with the diagram of the 11th century Chinese drawing. When the circle is full, they say that the feminine is beginning to move. I feel that this is an indication for our process.

---

## Drawing

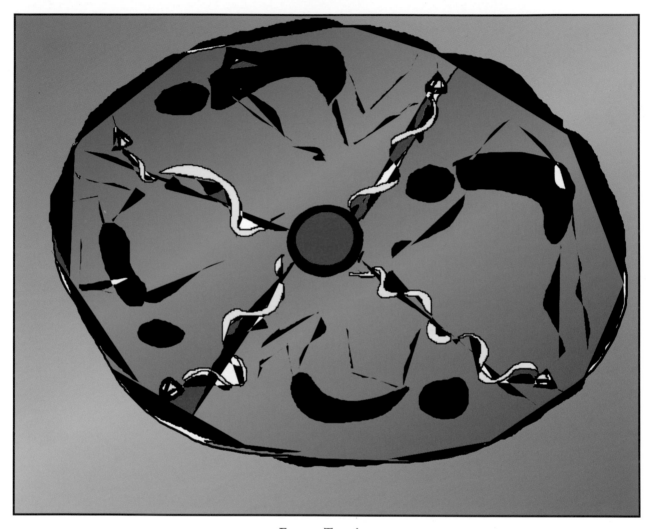

**Forces Turning**

She felt that something was moving within her. She could not define the forces that were turning around in her. This is the beginning of a movement.

### Tray 7
### Woman Age 46

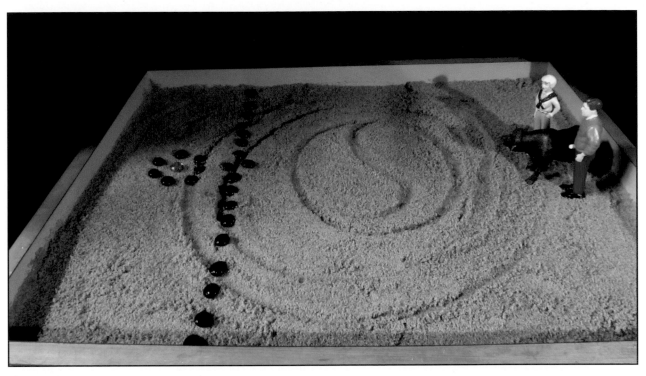

**Tray 7a**
**Woman Age 46**

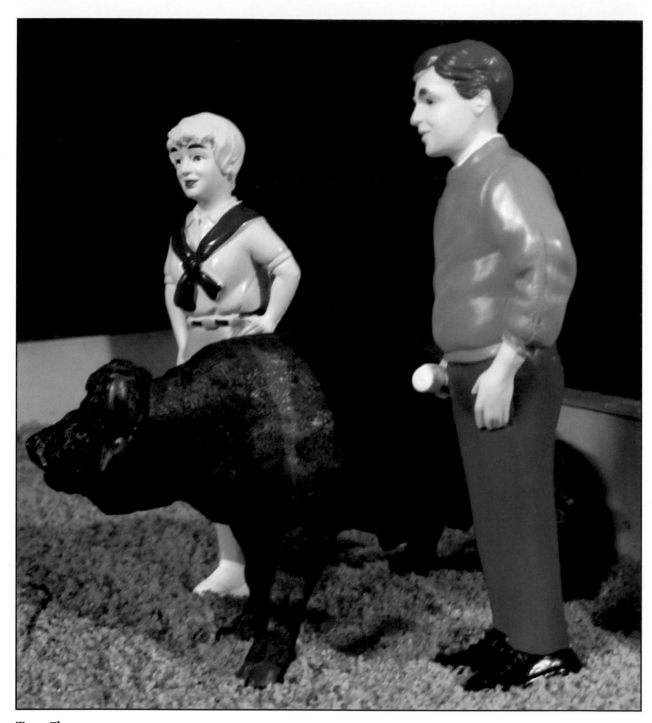

**Tray 7b**
**Woman Age 46**

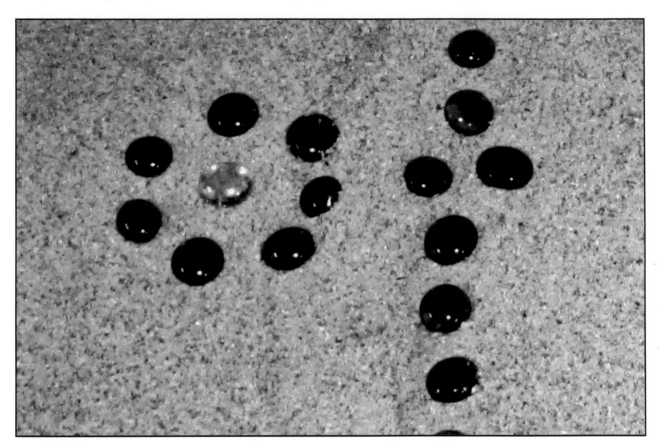

**Tray 7c**
**Woman Age 46**

A man and a woman have to guide the bull across the spiral.

In Zen there are the Ox Herding Pictures. There is the taming of the ox, of the negative forces. Here they are masculine forces. They are transforming and are being guided to the center. She felt that these forces she was feeling were so strong that they need masculine and feminine forces to guide them.

This is a wheel that begins to turn. It leads to a new phase that is displayed by the color red. Here is an indication of the fire element with the red. This could be a new development of the feeling function. She will guide these forces with the growing of the masculine and feminine sides of her own growing psyche.

The Ox Herding Pictures are about the taming of the mind. The ox is the mind. When the mind goes astray or is used in a negative way, we must control it and keep it in its total aspect. Here we have this expression of the totality she had before. Also the sand in this picture looks like a yin-yang. With the beginning of this movement it then goes up through all five elements.

**Tray 8**
**Woman Age 46**

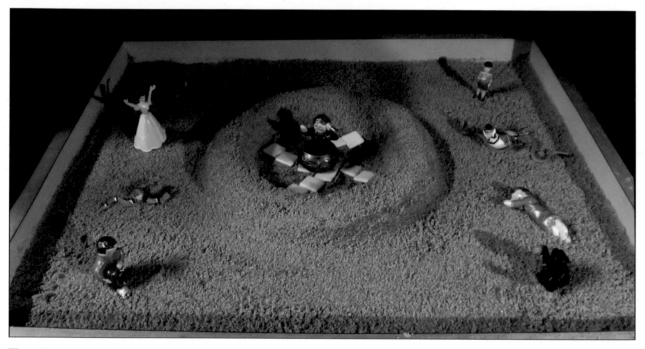

**Tray 8a**
**Woman Age 46**

**Drawing**

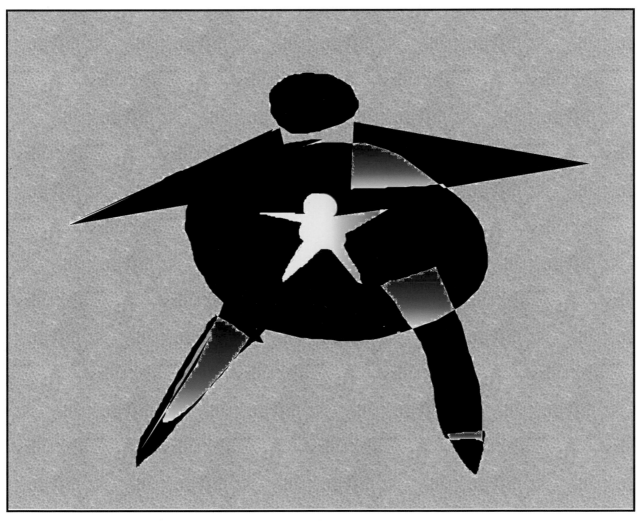

**With Dancing Shiva**

Now she sees herself as the five-pointed star. Last time it was on the bottom of the sea. Later it was the star of Bethlehem. Now it is herself. We can see how she began to feel more and more secure.

She got a letter from America saying to come home. I had to talk to her at this point, because things were so new for her. I thought she had such a strong experience that she could live with this.

## Drawing

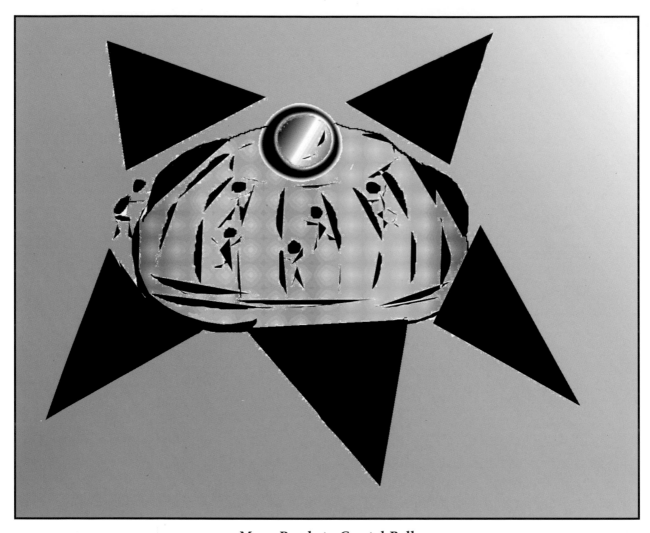

**Many Roads to Crystal Ball**

*This is a crystal ball with many roads and many people going up and down.*

Very often when people go through this deep experience, they get an inner wish to share it. There are many people coming up and down here. She wishes that many people can experience this.

## Drawing - Dream

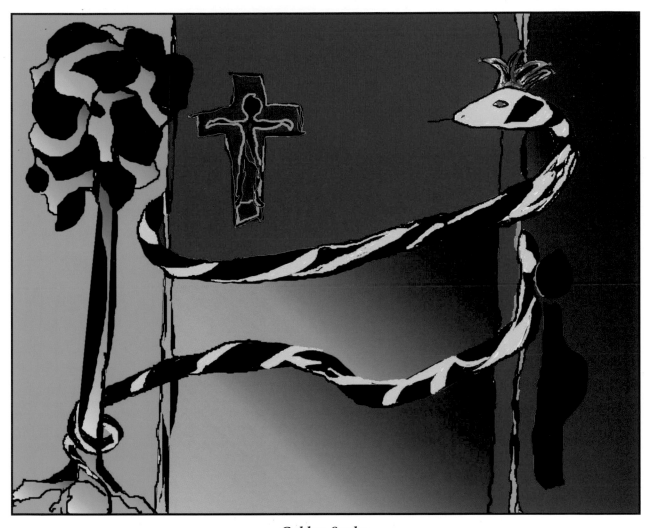

**Golden Snake**

*A tree, a golden snake and a pregnant woman*

## Drawing - Dream

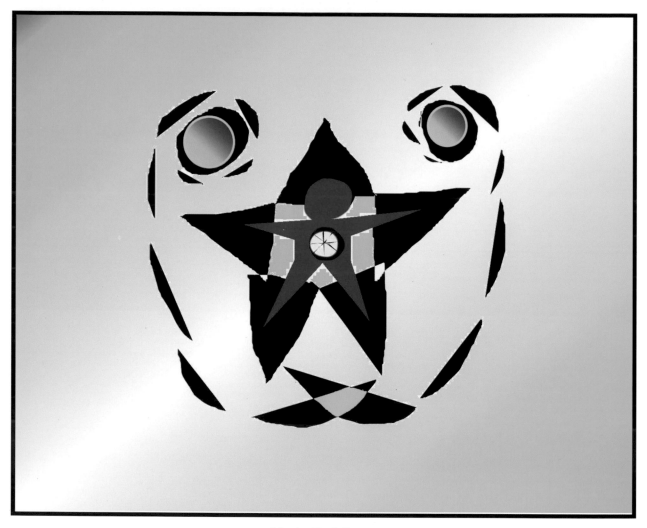

**Me in Red Dress**

This is her in a red dress.

**Tray 9**
**Woman 46**
**Final Tray**

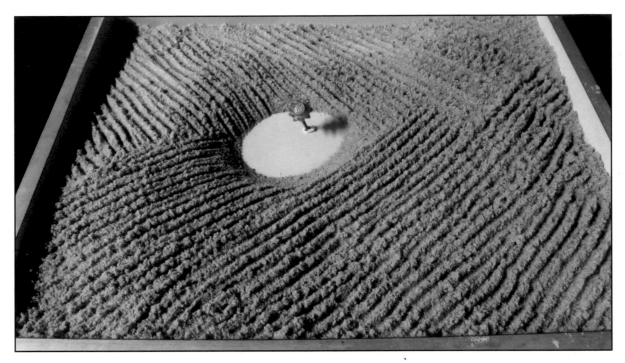

**Tray 9**
**Woman 46**

This is the earth being made ready for new life. When the water and earth come together the lotus begins to bloom. Remember what the boy said, *"Where the water and the earth meet, the white flower blooms and there is happiness."*

She went home and became a teacher. She worked in an under privileged area of town. She wrote and illustrated books for the children. She did beautiful artwork. She married again, happily this time. She has worked so hard. You see how this can happen when, *"...there is no other chance."*

**End**
**Woman 46**

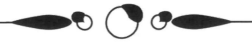

# 31 March – 2 April 1989

## *Carmel, California*

The depths in ourselves know what we do not know consciously. We touch the collective unconscious with sandplay. This shows us the path where we need to go. Sandplay facilitates the individuation process. In sandplay we become conscious of unconscious contents and integrate them into our lives.

When something happens inwardly and outwardly at the same time it is a *synchronistic* event. What is displayed with the symbols is a coming together of inner and outer happenings. This provides for the next step of development in the person. Thus, it is vital that we understand what is going on, not necessarily verbally, but with our intuition. When we see repeated images in the sand, we must ask what is going on. As soon as I grasp the client's unconscious situation, the images will change.

This inner understanding is known more in the Far East. Here we are trained to understand things consciously. No real transformation takes place in consciousness alone.

# Woman – Early 30's

## *Pregnant*

This case is of a dark-skinned mixed race, Latin woman, married to a Caucasian man from the same country. She was in her thirties and pregnant. I did not think it was a good idea to work with a pregnant woman, because she needs to be completely there for the growing child. The mother and the child need to have an intimate life that I did not think should be shared with someone outside. However, this client was so much in need I decided to work with her anyway. Here we will see images of the pregnancy and of the birth. This shows us that when we work in the sand, it always anticipates the actual fact.

This woman was from a farming family with eleven children. There were eight boys and three girls. She had a three year-old son of her own. She said that her mother loved the boys, but not the girls. The mother was white, and her father was of African descent. She had a graduate degree. She said that she suffered because she was the only dark-skinned student in the university and that she never felt good about that. She never felt fully accepted.

When she worked, she did so silently. She did not talk with me at all. Everything came through the sandplays. I have never had anyone who did not say a word, but she felt at ease with it. She had an initial dream that she shared, although we did not talk about it or analyze it.

**Dream**

> A dark woman gives me a dark fish, but when I cut open it is white inside.

Initial dreams will sometimes give us an overview of the analytical process.

In alchemy the *nigredo* is at the beginning and is followed by the *albedo*, the whitening. This is the clarification of a dark situation with which we originally come into the analytical, sandplay process. The alchemical process is the process of becoming gold. It is a process of purification. In Jung's work on alchemy, white is compared to the queen. Here the client said that the fish was white inside.

This may mean that she will change something in her feminine attitude. White means becoming more conscious about ourselves and our way of life.

We must accept that we have dark, unknown things in ourselves. Beyond the shadow in the true depths within ourselves we find an incredibly beautiful situation. This shows the totality of the personality without throwing a shadow. This is the Self, the total aspect within ourselves. Without any exceptions, we all have this. I remember one little three year-old child asking his baby brother, "*Tell me about God. I am beginning to forget.*" This is the secret for pure happiness. We must try to get in touch with this.

**Tray 1**
**Pregnant Woman**

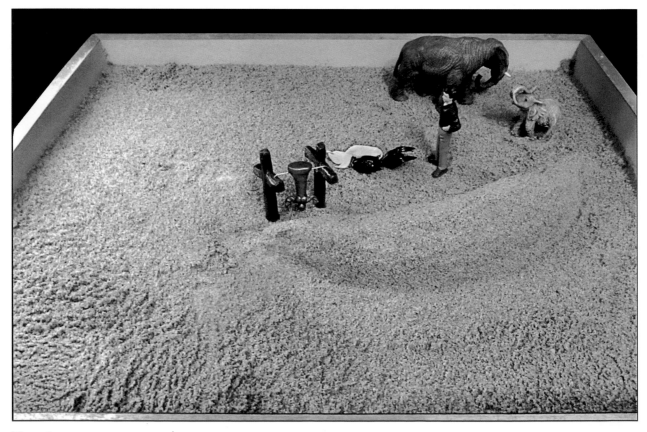

**Tray 1a**
**Pregnant Woman**

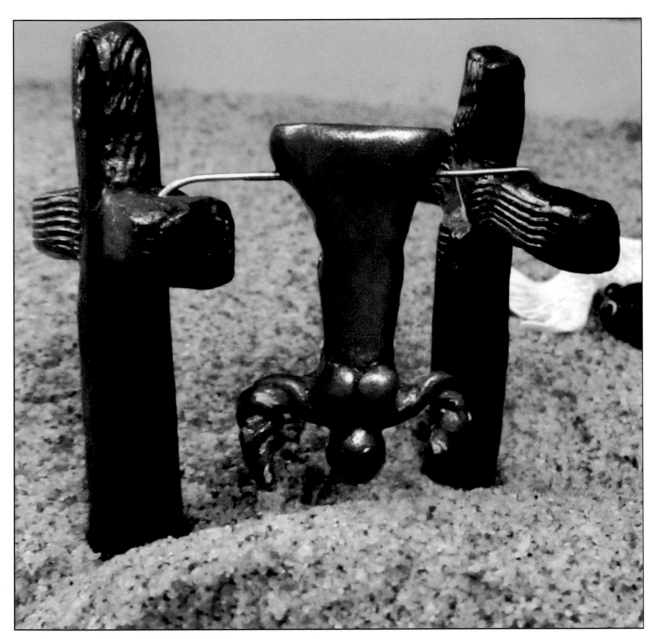

**Tray 1b**
**Pregnant Woman**

Initially this tray feels broken at the top, sad. There is nothing living, no greenery.

A woman, the goddess of Crete, is hanging between two crosses. Maybe this is the white, patriarchal culture that is so painful, the Christianity. She was Christian and lived in a white society that was predominated by rationalism and technology. This shows us that she is suffering from living with too much intellectualism. When St. Peter was crucified, he hung upside down because he did not feel worthy to hang upright. This is a betrayal of herself.

In the Tarot, the Hanging Man is about being able to see things from the other side.

A huge elephant is leaving and a young elephant is arriving. Maybe an old, heavy situation is leaving. The big load she has been carrying is leaving. Maybe something new and young is coming. Maybe she will be able to free herself from this burden.

The crescent moon is about change. Jung compared the individuation process to becoming a white, full moon, as a complete clarification of issues. Here some clarification is beginning to take place.

There are two fish, one dark and one light, being watched by a man. The issue of dark and light is a problem. Here the masculine side looks at this.

Here the Goddess of Crete is with two snakes in her hands. This is the earthy, warm quality of the feminine arising in her. Not only is there the question of the black and white, but also one of the feminine nature. It seems that the question is about living with her feminine qualities. Her mother did not accept her, but supported her brothers. Maybe she has not lived up to her feminine potentials. Her husband wanted her to continue her studies, but she wanted to be a mother. The elephants are strong, good mothers. They are also guides.

We see groups of twos here. This is a sign that something has to become conscious. It is still unconscious, but will soon become conscious. It is aiming toward consciousness.

**Tray 2**
**Pregnant Woman**

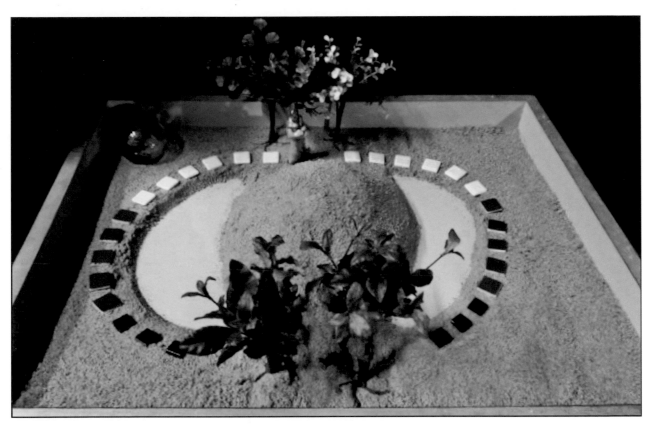

**Tray 2a**
**Pregnant Woman**

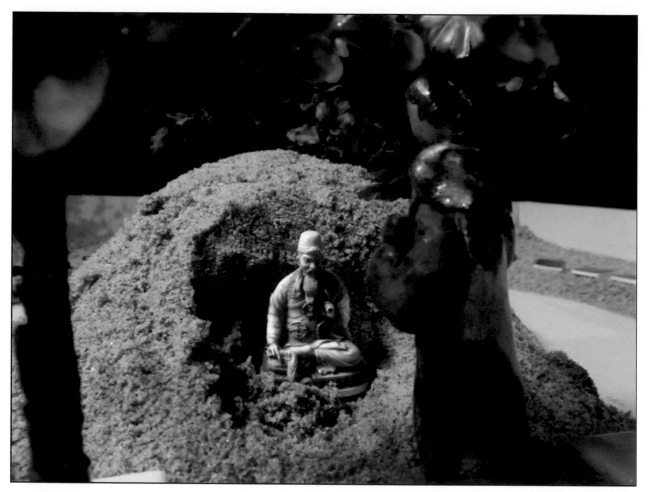

**Tray 2b**
**Pregnant Woman**

Here there are autumn trees in the front and green trees in the back. This is like the elephants. One goes away and the other is coming. The more conscious life is near the foreground, and the less known things are farther away.

There is a cave with a wise man in it. She said that the wise man gave the woman in blue a lapis lazuli. This is a very precious stone that combines many chemicals together. This is like the philosopher's stone in alchemy. In ancient Egypt the kings lined their helmets with lapis, because they thought it helped them communicate with the heavens. Blue reminds us of the cloak of Mary. This gift is given to her from within the womb, the cave, the darkest, most secret place. We must get in contact with the darkness.

Jung said that it is there that the light shines the brightest. Here she finds something very valuable in her darkness. We can see that in the darkness of herself, she will find her own precious stone.

The wise man has a numinous quality. This must be so to have the experience of the Self. This is why she chose this wise man.

The stepping stones become yellow and red as they move toward the green trees. This is a renewal that comes out of the darkest place. Red is fire, love and feeling. Maybe she has not really experienced real love so far. Maybe her Christianity has not helped her experience real love. When she is able to accept the black with the same value as the white, then she will be whole. We cannot reject our dark side.

The glass ball is a totality. It is a union of opposites, but here it is on the side in the corner. It is not in the center yet, but it is somewhere.

This is like an island. It may still be a feeling of isolation. There is isolation when you go alone. We deal with these problems alone. The free and protected space provides a place for the client to follow her own path.

**Tray 3**
**Pregnant Woman**

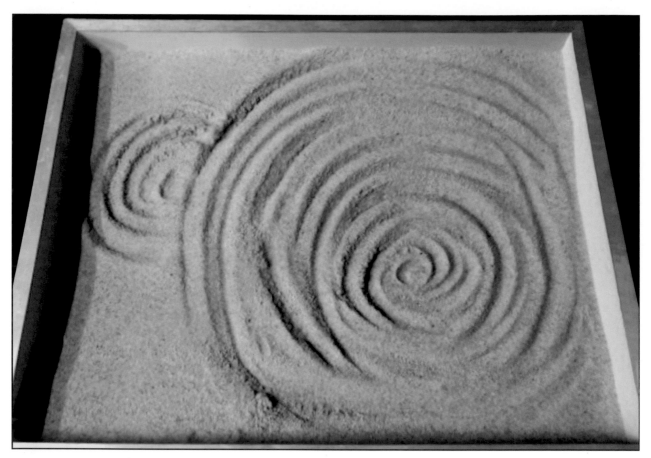

**Tray 3**
**Pregnant Woman**

This is dry sand. I felt that this was like a whirlpool. Something was working that would take her into the depths. We see here the necessity for her to go within to deeper levels. Here I think she felt drawn to her unconscious.

**Tray 4**
**Pregnant Woman**

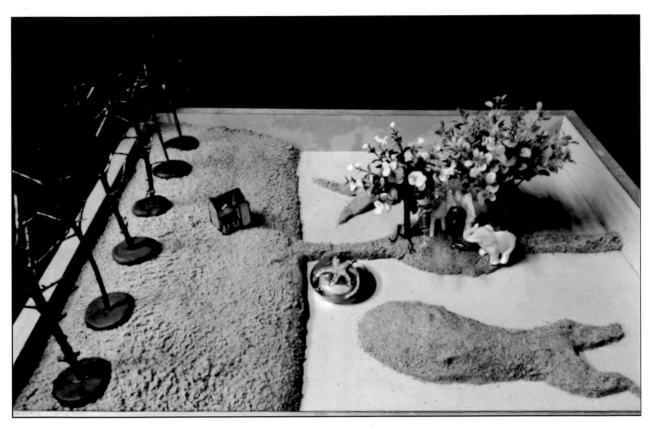

**Tray 4a**
**Pregnant Woman**

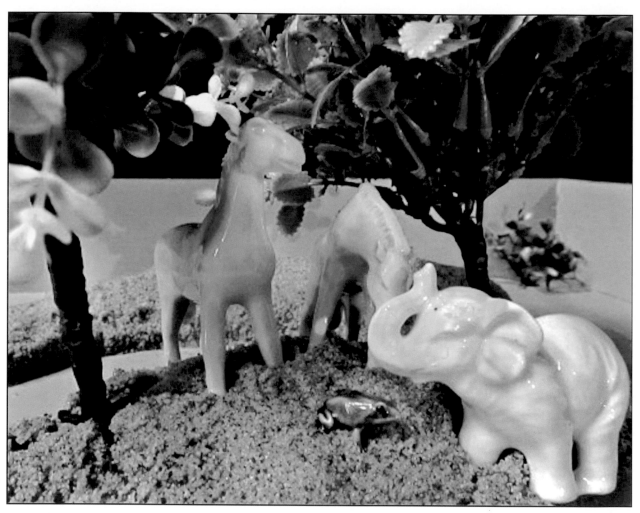

**Tray 4b**
**Pregnant Woman**

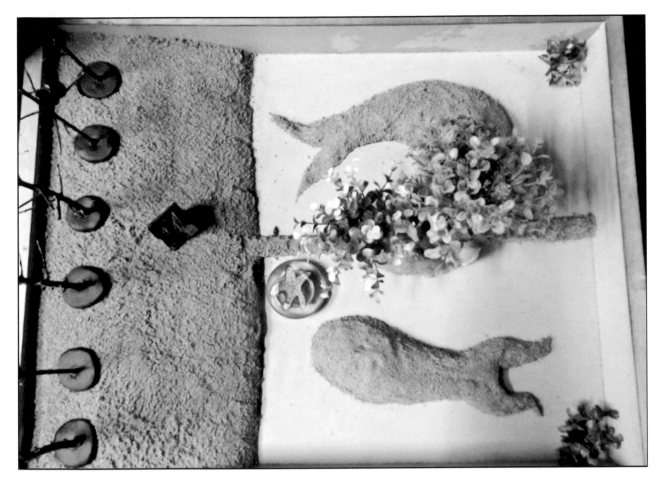

**Tray 4c**
**Pregnant Woman**

This was the tray during which she told me she was pregnant.

One side refers to the conscious side where she feels that something is dead, not working any more. The left side is barren and burned. This is how she felt. The right side begins to come alive and is two thirds of the picture. This is just as in the last tray where the whirlpool took two thirds of the tray. Watch these processes from tray to tray. The psyche takes what is important from the prior picture and develops it. The dead trees indicate that her situation is bad on the outside, but inside she carries new life. But penetrating into the unconscious, the water, there is a little island. The island is in the center of the water, the unconscious. This could indicate a new birth, the symbol of what is growing within her. She said that the animals were still sleeping.

The white animals often indicate a connection with the divine quality. The white elephant is the creator of Buddha. It is said that the mother of the Buddha had a dream that a white elephant came in her window, encircled here three times and disappeared into her right side. This is seen as the pre-incarnation of the Buddha - an animal with a divine quality. Buddha was born out of the side of his mother. Two trays ago, the woman went to see the wise man. Perhaps this was as the mother of Buddha did to find out she was expecting a savior.

There is a form of Tibetan Buddhist meditation that begins with a dark elephant. Progressively through the meditation the elephant becomes white. When the elephant is white, this means you have reached perfect concentration.

The white horses are associated with the Christ, Buddha and Mohammed. This island shows the Self, but she said that these animals are asleep. This is the part of the unconscious that she is touching and it is not yet awake. Her conscious side has not fulfilled her, so she looks into the unconscious. But it is not awake yet.

There is also a little frog on the island. The frog has to do with transformation. It is born as a pollywog. In the fairy tale of the frog king the frog is the preliminary form of the human being. It can become more than it has lived up to until this point. This is a preliminary Self that lies dormant in her. Every now and then we see a small frog appear in the early pictures. This can be an indication of a baby coming.

Here are two fish swimming in the water. This is the contents of the unconscious and the symbol of Christ. In Greek this is *ICTUS,* which means *Christ the Son of God the Savior.* So here we have a deep religious image of her inner beliefs. This reminds us of the two crosses in the first tray. In *Aion,* Jung says the fish that goes from the land down means that something moves from the spiritual to the material. The fish that comes from the water up to the land brings the spirit to the earth.

There is a piece of sea glass with a star on it. This becomes meaningful to her. This is a circular form with a star on it. Stars reflect ancient light. As a star that has been in the water for so long, (sea glass aging) this must have to do with something that takes a long time. Her Self has been dormant all of this time. Maybe this means that this sandplay needs a lot of time, a lot of washing clean.

**Tray 5**
**Pregnant Woman**

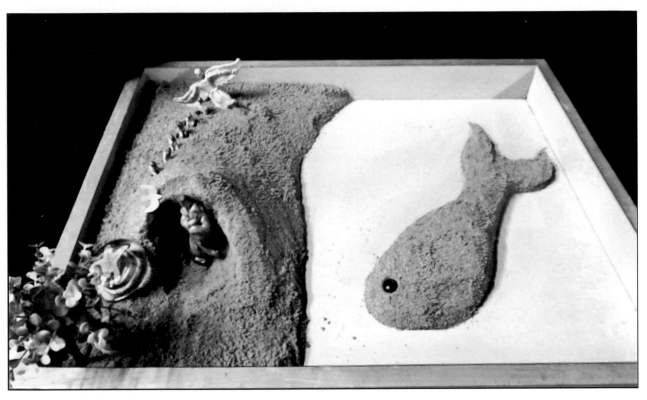

**Tray 5a**
**Pregnant Woman**

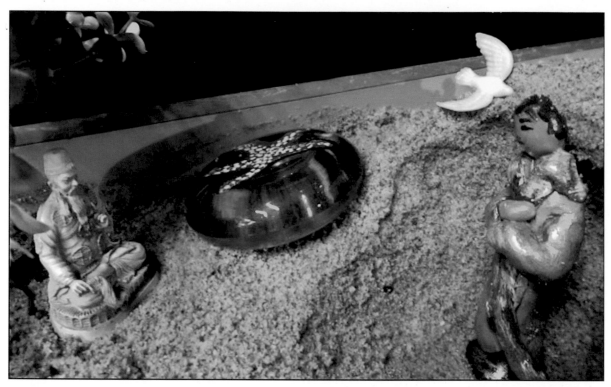

**Tray 5b**
**Pregnant Woman**

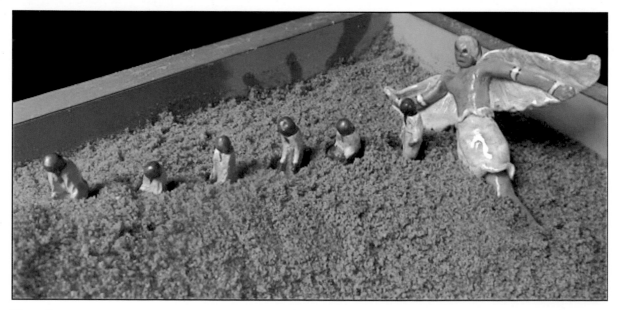

**Tray 5c**
**Pregnant Woman**

Here there are six dark men without hair. She poked holes in the sand as if to plant the men. She said it was a ritual that was done in the evening. They are planting seed into the ground. Putting seed into the ground is an act of fertility.

These men are all bald. Hair has to do with thought, with something that grows out of our thinking. Now they have lost all of that. There was too much rationality, and the masculine side had to change. She lived under masculine control. Here the men are without hair, because she needs something else. This would be the putting of seed into the earth. This quality had to bow down to the earth, to touch the earth with the head. From the feminine ground, something new can grow. Shaving the head is an act of humbling oneself. This work needs a certain humility. Icarus flew too high up and melted his wings. Then he fell back to the earth. Being humble and accepting something that comes from below is important.

The fish is swimming toward the cave - before we had two fish. One was going down and the other was coming up. This fish aims toward the cave. This is about insemination, the coming together of the masculine and the feminine. It is about conception.

The woman here wears blue and the fish has a red eye. The red-eyed fish aims toward the cave where the blue is dominant. Maybe the red and the blue have to come together. Jung said that blue had to do with the thinking function, and the red with feeling. This is a fertilization of love toward the thinking side. Here we see something that has to come together.

The wise man under the tree is present with all of the things that happen. There is the fertilization of the earth with these men. All together there are six men plus Icarus. The prior tray had six burned trees. Here we have six bald men who go to the earth to get new energy. She poked holes to plant them. This is a new planting in her unconscious. The earth has been dead and infertile. Here we see it being inseminated.

Now there is a white dove. When Noah was on the ark, it was the dove that brought the twig indicating that they had found land. This is an aspect of the spiritual side. This goes together with the woman in the blue coat. This is the descent of the Holy Spirit, the annunciation. This is another image of coming together. And the coming together of the red and the white is a new birth.

**Tray 6**
**Pregnant Woman**

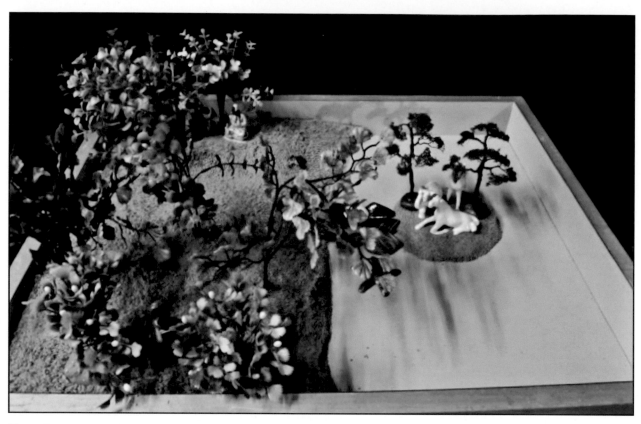

**Tray 6a**
**Pregnant Woman**

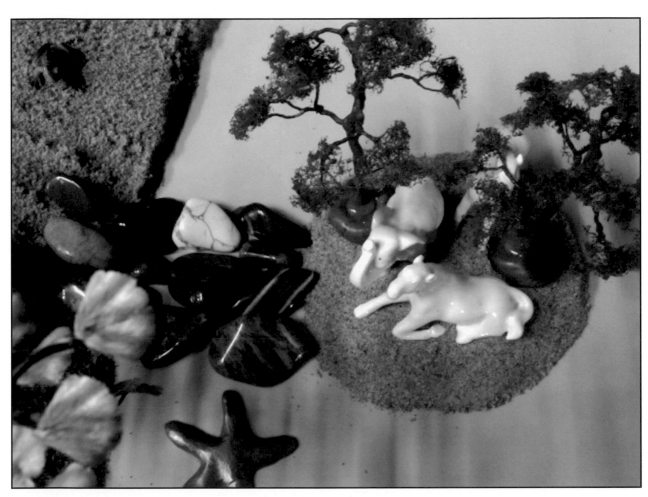

**Tray 6b**
**Pregnant Woman**

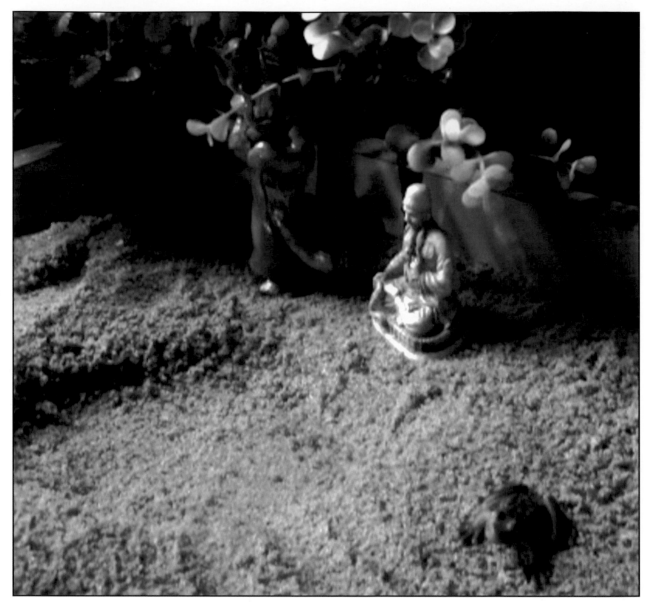

**Tray 6c**
**Pregnant Woman**

Before, the men put seeds in the earth. Now we see a lot of growth.

Here there are three lines that connect the little island. This is a further indication of the pregnancy, as there are three blood vessels in the umbilical cord that connect the child to the mother. We see here that her inner spiritual side is growing at the same time her child is growing.

Now the frog has crossed over to the mainland. This is a pre-figuration of the prince. Perhaps she begins, here on a lower level, (frog, water, earth) to bring a new masculine quality into life. He is on the way.

The wise man and the woman are together. He is her guide for this process.

The masculine side, the animus, is very insecure and uncertain. She begins to feel that all she has learned in school, etc., is not what she thought it was. The men whose heads are bowed have moved from a position of arrogance to re-thinking everything. As there is so much greenery in this tray, we see that she is moving toward a more natural side of herself.

So we see the baby growing in her and the possibility of a psychological change in her. Many aspects develop at the same time.

If you do sandplay during pregnancy, you will have the most beautiful baby!

## Tray 7
## Pregnant Woman

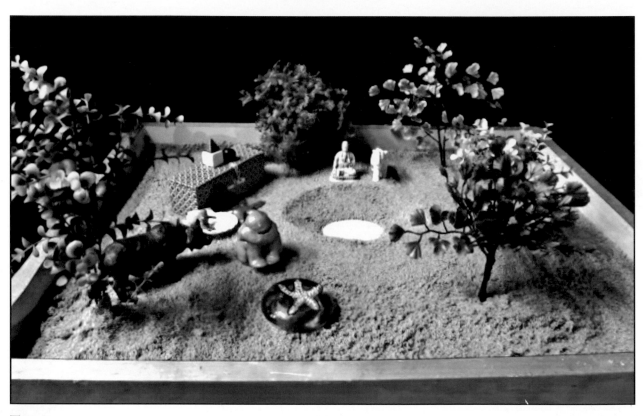

**Tray 7a**

**Pregnant Woman**

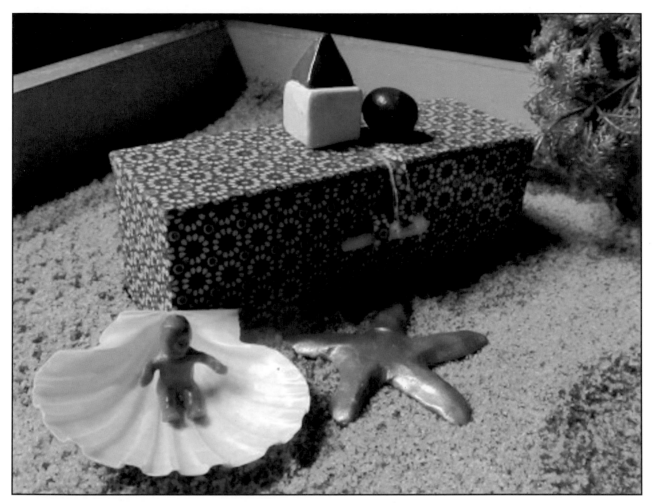

**Tray 7b**
**Pregnant Woman**

*This is a box and in this box is a treasure that no one has seen for many years.*

This box contains something that has not been seen in a long time. The treasure box and the shell each hold something that is becoming. This is her own birth of the Self and the baby that is coming. The shell has a feminine quality. In Japan, when a woman is pregnant, she often receives a shell with a pearl in it as a sign of the fulfillment of her womanhood. This is here, but not yet visible.

Both sides come together now, the land and the island. Here are the elements fire, the triangle; earth, the box; and water, the sphere. The elements, earth, water and fire are present. These are the three basic elements by which the human body exists. Eastern medicine uses the five elements. When the five elements are in harmony, then the body is healthy. Air and spirit are still missing here. The sea star next to the three elements shows that there are five elements for a fulfillment. Perhaps the spirit is in the wise man, but air is missing. There is too much air in the pondering man. The man who is holding his head is the masculine side that is beginning to know what is happening. It is as if he is asking, "*...where am I and what am I doing?*" She has to sacrifice a little of his intellect.

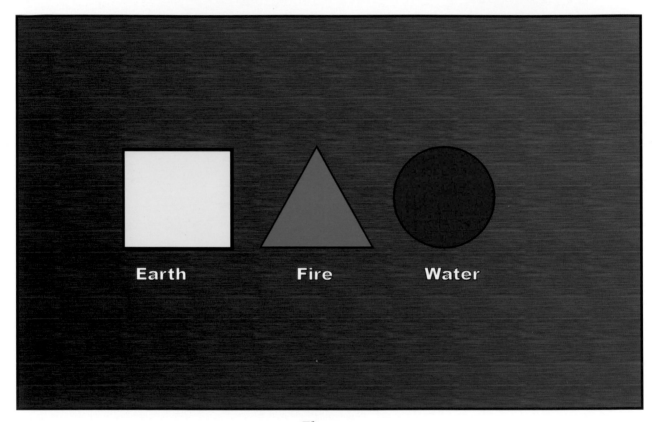

**Elements**

The ox works very hard. In the Zen *Ox Herding Pictures*, the mind is wandering about, untamed. You have to tame the mind to make it available to help with integration. With this ox, it seems that there is still a task to do. There is something that she still had to learn and to exercise it. Once she gets in touch with this, she will become more complete. This also shows a path toward consciousness, toward enlightenment. The ox is next to the star, which may indicate the fulfillment of the totality. The star is the energy of the tamed mind.

The wise man is a guide that has a more developed mind. Together with the white elephant, he has this divine quality. There is an inner peace, a contentment in this picture. Through this place there is the possibility of new growth. The cave of the womb from the last tray and the little island seem to have come together here.

---

## The Zen Ox Herding Pictures

The Zen Ox Herding Pictures are an allegory of the struggle with the conscious position to subordinate itself to the Self. The ten pictures recount the struggle a man undergoes in his attempt to catch and herd the ox back home. There are many depictions of this story. These ink drawings are by Tensho Shubun, Japanese Zen Buddhist monk and painter from the fifteenth century. The pictures are presented in two columns of five in series from the top down.

1. In Search of the Bull - Aimless Searching
2. Discovery of the Footprints - Discovery of the Path
3. Perceiving the Bull - Only the Rear and Not its Head
4. Catching the Bull - Great Struggle with Many Escapes
5. Taming the Bull - Less Struggle - Bull Becomes Gentle and Obedient
6. Riding the Bull Home - Great Joy
7. The Bull Transcended - Once Home, the Bull is Forgotten - Stillness
8. Bull and Self Transcended - All Empty
9. Reaching the Source - Unconcerned Within and Without
10. Return to the Marketplace - Spreading Enlightenment

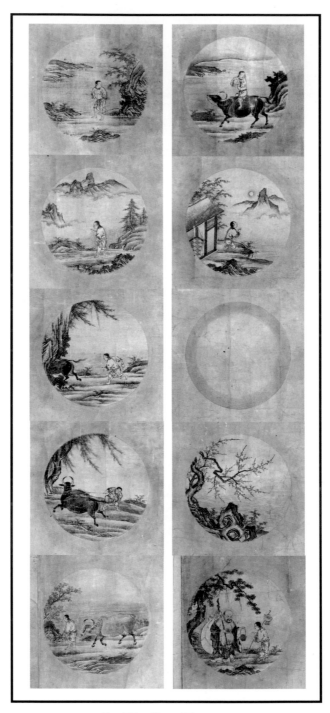

**Ox Herding Pictures**
*Tensho Shubun, 15th c*

**Tray 8**
**Pregnant Woman**

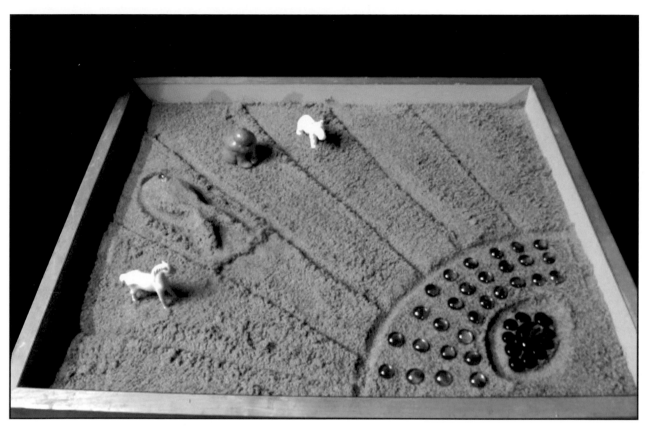

**Tray 8a**
**Pregnant Woman**

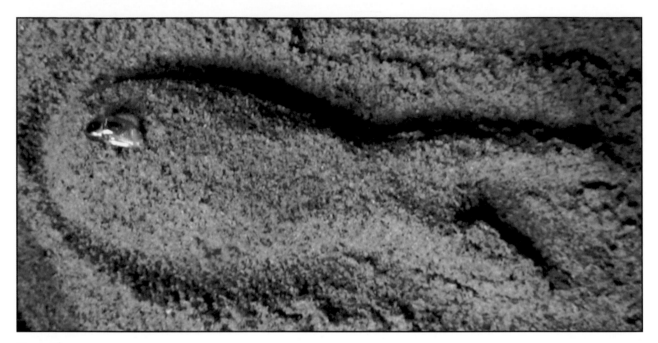

**Tray 8b**
**Pregnant Woman**

This could be an eye, or one quarter of the sun. This shows the divine aspect coming. She is seeing it. There are seven rays and seven rows of three stones. There are two rows of four stones. The four is about completeness, and the three is about being on the way. There is a dynamism between the three and four and between the red and blue. This is the thinking and the feeling functions coming together.

If we see it as an eye, maybe this means there is a possibility of becoming more conscious of this. We have seven rays and four figures. The masculine, three, and the feminine, four, are beginning to make peace.

The white elephant and the white horse look toward this eye, or sun, and so does the pondering man. The negative influence of too much intellectualism is still here.

This fish has a yellow eye. This is a new color. A new aspect is growing out of the union of the red and the blue. Yellow is the sun, warmth, light and clarity. It has to do with the intuitive function. Here this may be a spiritual inspiration. I think that this fish is swimming in a new direction which will bring some new elements.

The fish shows the value of the unconscious from which new elements can come up. This is why it appears as a prominent symbol for her. In addition, her experience with Christianity is an issue for her. The intellect and nature have been in conflict within her. The birth of the child is another issue, and there is the issue of being black and white.

## Tray 9
## Pregnant Woman

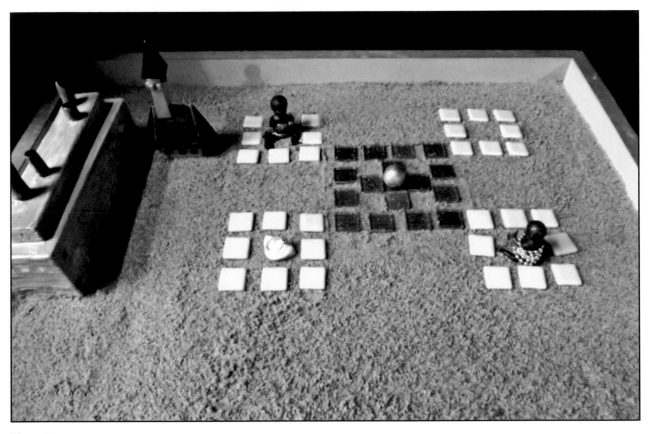

**Tray 9a**
**Pregnant Woman**

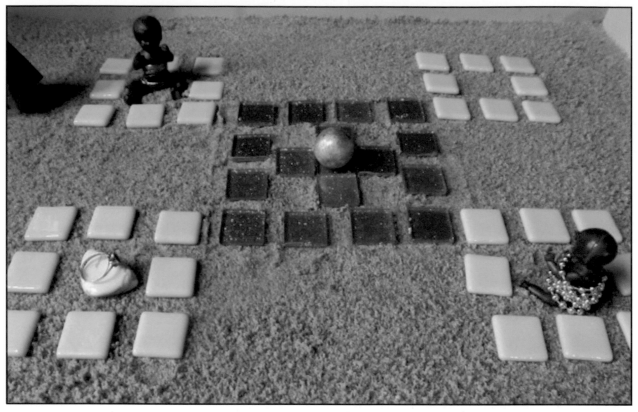

**Tray 9b**
**Pregnant Woman**

She said that this is her father's factory. When you walk through it you come to a church. And behind the church is a garden that no one has seen before. She came to the garden through the way of her father. She had a good relationship with the father, although her mother did not like the girls. So we see it was her relationship with her father that gave her the religious possibility. She said that her happiest day was when her father took her to school for the first time. Her father was rich through nature. He had large ranches.

This was the first time that she realized that she would get to something important in herself. Her father had already died. He left her a small house, which he loved very much.

The four squares in the garden are made of three-sided walls. This is the movement toward wholeness. The empty square is something new to come. The garden is a precious enclosure. It is a safe place – a symbol of the Self.

There is great value in this garden. The gold cross may show a different value of religion than she had before. The two babies are also encircled with the great value of gold. Through this experience she may be able to accept the darkness as a value. This is very important to her.

The number five appears here in the five squares. This was also seen in the sea star and the five elements that were to be found. Her fulfillment can be found through the gift of nature that her father gave her. He is the dark parent. Behind the factory was the church. And behind the church was the garden that has not been seen. What is dark now becomes of great value.

With the degree of concentration seen in the last tray, we can expect that this emphasis on the masculine and self-derision cannot continue. We expect that a movement will come out of this.

We are always on the path. We are never at the end. Every moment of silence may contain the original sadness which is the loss of the primordial Self we had at birth. Here the two black babies are shown with great value. We must remember the beginning of the whole story where she was hanged between two crosses.

Perhaps her life was like a mission where Catholicism was forced on the native people. Perhaps she begins to see things from an inner perspective now. Remember the Hanging Man in the Tarot, which says that we must see things in a different way.

The golden cross here in the garden is equally long on each side. Yellow was introduced in the last tray in the eye of the fish.

The ring on the white stone announces her being. And the empty square is the further development that she does not yet see. She is on the path and not at the end. There are still new things to come.

## Tray 10
## Pregnant Woman

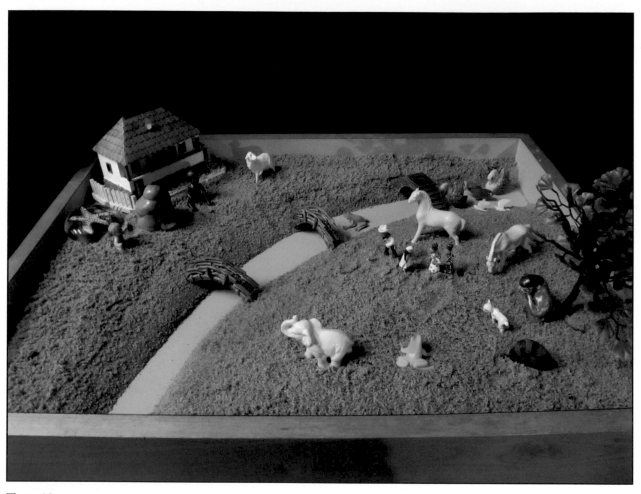

**Tray 10a**
**Pregnant Woman**

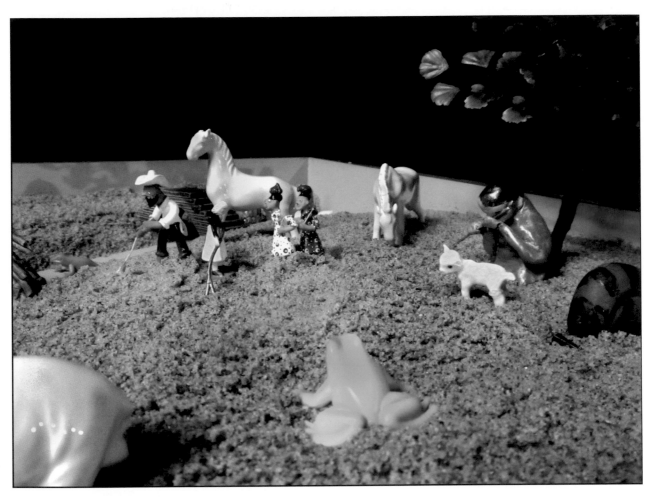

**Tray 10b**
**Pregnant Woman**

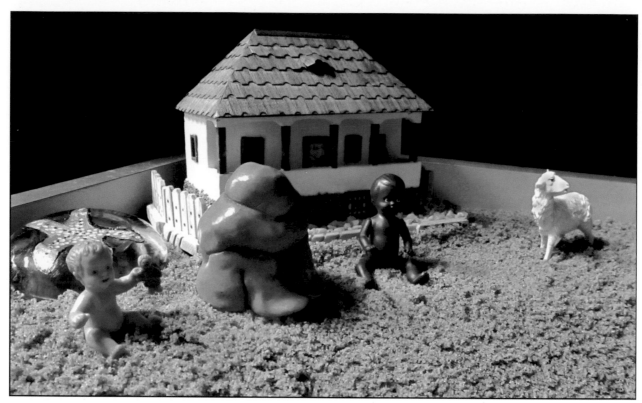

**Tray 10c**
**Pregnant Woman**

Here we see many groups of threes and fours. Three is dynamic, and four is more of an achievement. It is an aspect of the totality. Before this has been a theme, but not shown with human beings. Here it is with three women and one man. This shows greater integration.

There are two babies and the dark and the light have equal value. First she gave the dark the value with the jewelry and the thread. Now a new dimension opens up with an equal value to white and black. This is not in her consciousness, but is preparing itself on a deeper level.

The four people are working. They are on the move.

There are three bridges with a frog in the middle of the river. It can also jump and make the connection between the two sides. Perhaps he is the fourth bridge. There is a snail on the edge of things, slowly coming in from the side. The snail is at home wherever he goes. The spiral shell is an indication of the path. This is the individuation process. The Aztecs saw the spiral as conception, gestation and birth. This reveals her pregnancy. There are two frogs here. One is between two bridges. The other frog is next to the snail. Maybe this frog helps this development that is indicated in the snail. The frog is an image of the new developing masculinity.

There is a baby lamb with the mother sheep on the other side of the river. This is a separation. There is not yet a very good feminine quality developed in her. The little lamb runs in the direction of his mother. This is a coming together. Here a new development in her feminine quality is getting prepared.

There is an active man on one side and a pondering man on the other. This is a new activity in the masculine. Up until now the masculine was giving her trouble, pondering about all of the difficulties. Here he works the ground. He is with nature and works with the feminine earth.

It is a great mistake to think that what is happening in the tray is already happening in the person. This is why interpretation is premature. These images are made from deeper levels of the unconscious. To interpret them takes them away from their own development on a deeper level. When I did interpret, I observed that the process did not continue. We can trust that what is shown in the image will become conscious and be integrated into the daily life. We must have this trust.

If a tray shows a current situation, interpretation is still not appropriate, as they are not aware of what the situation is. There is a loss with interpretation, because there is so much more in the unconscious than we can put into words. I have seen that when I try to talk about the situation, it disappears in the following trays.

In dreams, we give interpretation and in sandplay we do not. Sandplay comes from a deeper level than the dreams. An analyst in Europe worked once a week with sandplay and once with dreams. He told me he could clearly see that there were two different developments taking place on two different levels.

The carp in the river swims against the stream, indicating perseverance, carrying through. This shows that she will carry through.

Here are two swans. Sometimes they are seen as a symbol of the Self. Their necks are masculine and their bodies are feminine. In this respect it is a union of the opposites in itself. With the white color it can be seen as an image of the total aspect of the Self.

There are also two white doves. These are more natural and indicate a spiritual side.

**Tray 11**
**Pregnant Woman**

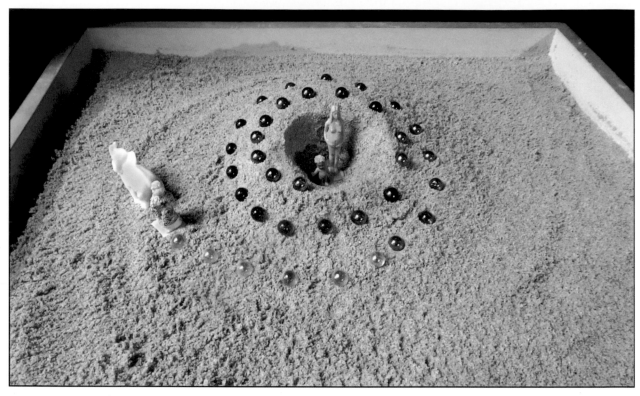

**Tray 11a**
**Pregnant Woman**

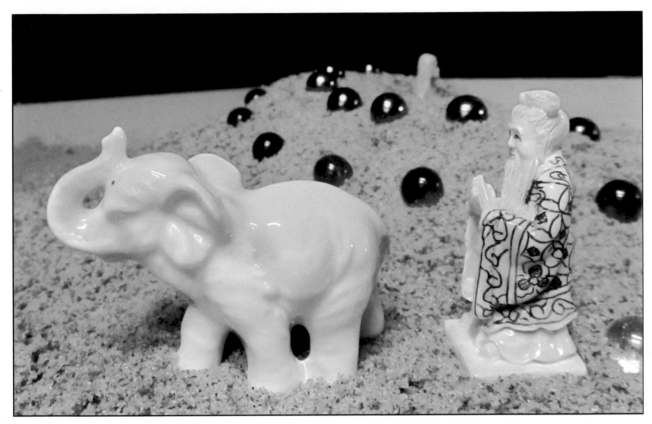

**Tray 11b**
**Pregnant Woman**

Here there are dark marbles going to light with a mother and child in the center. This is the first time we see the mother-child unity. Before they have been separated. We saw the spiral before on the snail. Here it is more developed. This is a pregnancy and a pregnancy of her new development. The marbles become lighter at the end of the spiral. This indicates the process of becoming conscious. They are guided out of the darkness by the wise man and the white elephant. This is the pregnancy of a divine quality. This indicates the actual birth process, and the birth within herself.

Here the white elephant encircles the mother of the divine, just as the white elephant encircled the mother of Buddha.

### *Participant Question*

*Regarding the choice to do this process with the woman while pregnant, under what circumstances it is not advisable?*

Had she been doing shadowy trays at the beginning of her process, I would have stopped it. But here she is getting in touch with her whole Self. There could be nothing better than this when pregnant. Now I know that women can be completely themselves while pregnant and doing sandplay.

### Tray 12
### Pregnant Woman

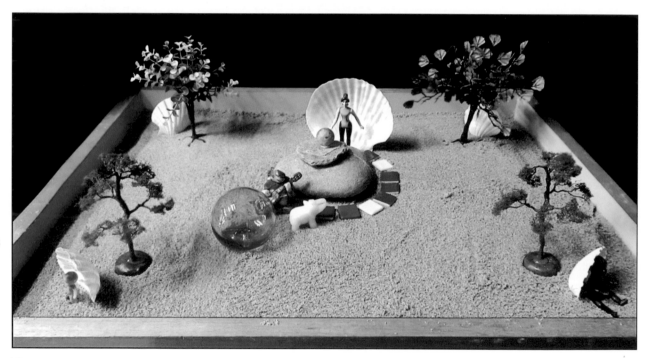

**Tray 12a**
**Pregnant Woman**

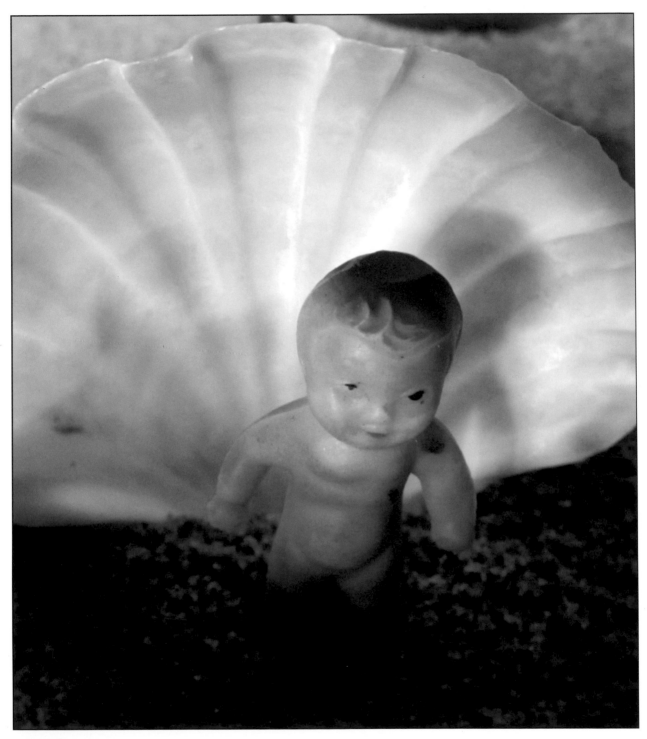

**Tray 12b**
**Pregnant Woman**

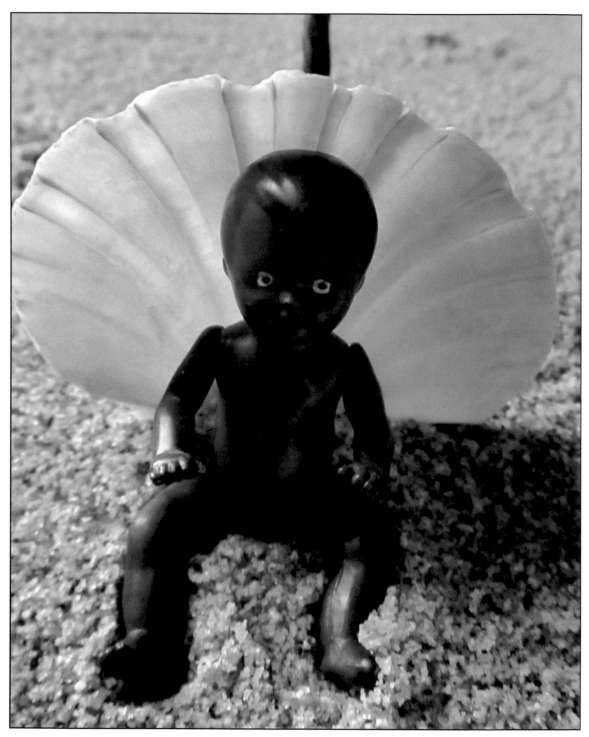

**Tray 12c**
**Pregnant Woman**

Here the man and the woman are shown together for the first time. This is a union of the masculine and the feminine for the first time as people. Now there is a balance between the masculine and the feminine. The center stones look like a breast. This is a female element beginning to have its influence. So this brings out the man and the woman as real human beings.

The woman is being born out of a shell. This is a reference to Venus. The man is now active. He is no longer the pondering man. The red color is important in the tiles. They are now connected with love and feeling. The man playing the guitar is connected to the feminine, and is no longer an overpowering masculine.

The shells are the feminine quality from the sea. Love plays an essential role here for the first time, as does nourishment through the breast.

The golden orb that was in the center of the cross is now here in the center of the breast. And the glass ball has moved more toward the center.

There are four babies. Two are black and two are white. There is an equal valuation to each now. Each is sheltered by the shells, the feminine side.

The main thing here is the appearance of this goddess of love. This has an influence on her masculine quality. Up until now the masculine was just pondering and was not really there.

This is a constellation of the Self. Notice that new developments usually evolve out of the center.

## Tray 13
## Pregnant Woman

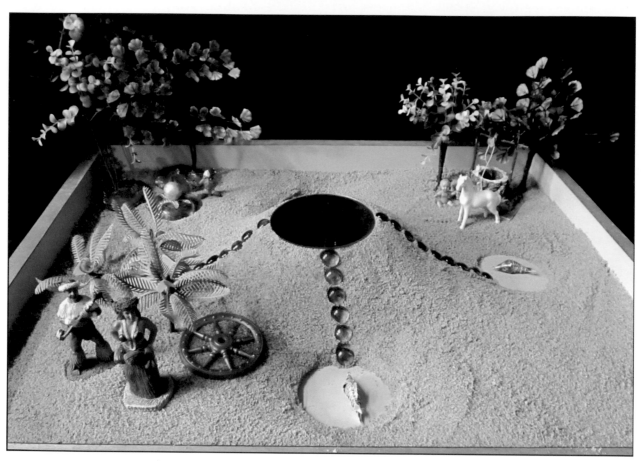

**Tray 13a**
**Pregnant Woman**

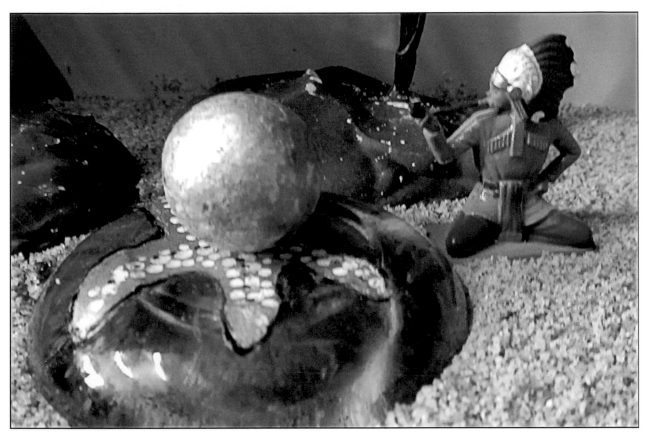

**Tray 13b**
**Pregnant Woman**

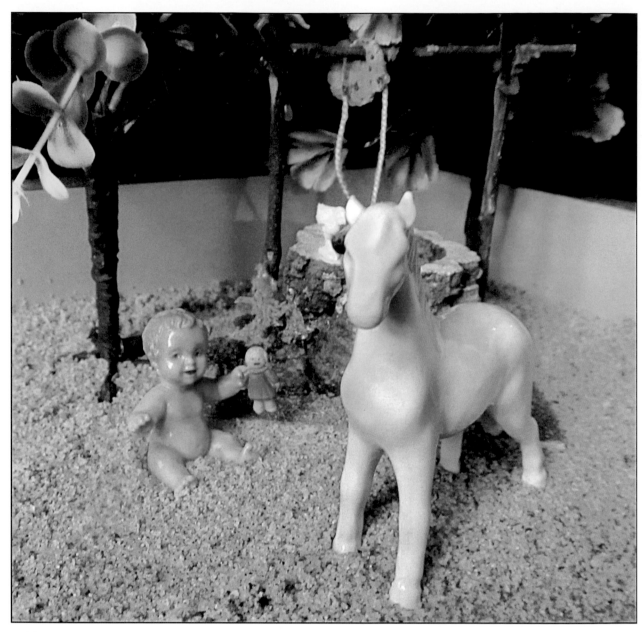

**Tray 13c**
**Pregnant Woman**

She calls this *paradise*. I showed this case to Stanislav Grof. He said that when the baby feels good and protected in the womb, it is like a paradisiacal situation. Here there are four streams that go to the four directions. They flow from paradise and nourish the world.

I felt that this was the beginning of the birth process. At this point she was seven months pregnant. I felt that this could be the first stage of the four states of birth. This is also a divine birth.

The mirror at the top of the mountain mirrors the sky. This is a union of heaven and earth. Mirrors usually indicate a way of becoming conscious. When you look into the mirror you see yourself. This is a pre-conscious situation, which is at a point of becoming conscious. This is an inner security that gives her the security for her own birth that is taking place.

The Indian with the peace pipe smokes the pipe after the war. And the eight-spoke wheel came after the enlightenment of Buddha. It began to turn in the opposite direction to help the world. It is a symbol of totality, or wholeness.

The well and the white horse make a divine situation. You can get the water out from the depths. This indicates that this comes from the very depths of herself. She feels peace in the depths of herself. There is a numinous quality here. She described the baby by the well as a divine child. This divine child is taken care of by this white horse, an animal that has a divine quality. This divine birth takes place at the *coniunctio*. (The union of opposites) It is a divine place. Thus there is no masculine or feminine involved. Of course, this is an anticipation of her own actual birth.

The dance and the musician are the joy and harmony. She now lives in more harmony between the masculine and the feminine. This could be with her husband as well as with an inner harmony. The Indians and the Hawaiians are so close to nature and the instincts. This is much different than the original over-valuation of the rational quality.

Grof speaks about the first day of birth as still a paradisiacal situation. But we know that there is an expelling from paradise, so we must pay attention to what comes next. We will have to see situations which are fearful and near death, like those that the mother and the baby go through during birth. Feelings of joy and of death are mixed during birth.

## Tray 14
## Pregnant Woman

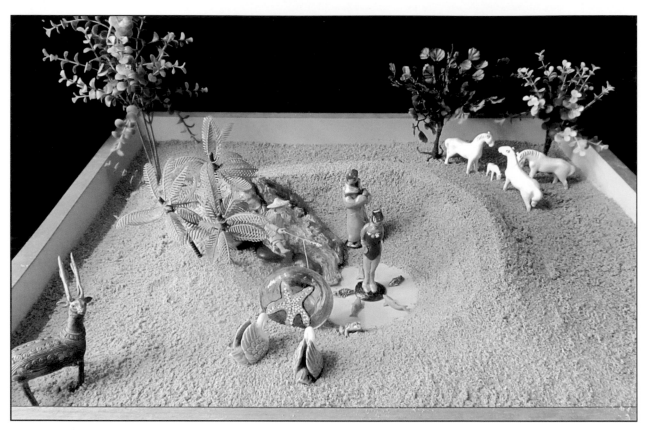

**Tray 14a**

**Pregnant Woman**

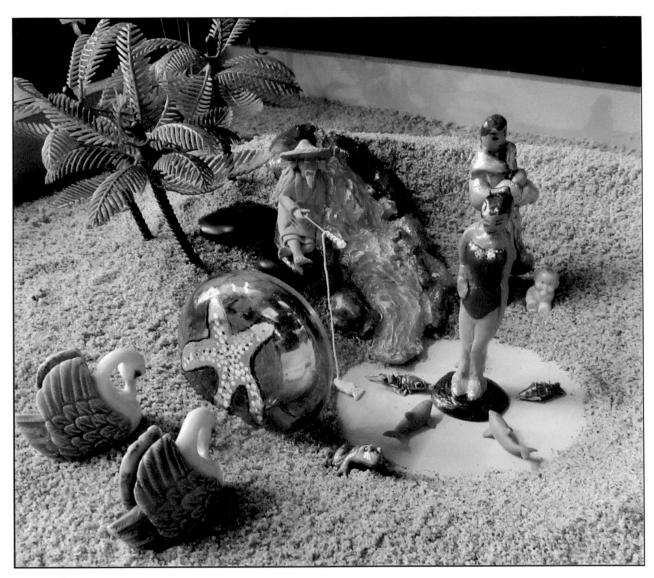

**Tray 14b**
**Pregnant Woman**

Here a woman, a young girl, appears out of the lake. This is a young woman who discovers her body and wants to show it off. Perhaps she felt a new birth within herself as a young woman – a renewed attitude toward the feminine. The woman with the blue coat watches the emergence of this young woman. She has the beginning of a new understanding.

There are three dolphins here. They have the capacity to get in and out of the water.

The mother and the baby are a preliminary image of the birth that will take place.

Here is a fisherman with a line down to the water. This is the masculine that begins to fish out of the unconscious, instead of moving up to his head. It is very interesting that the masculine begins to change and to reach into the depths.

The three horses surrounding the small horse may be the fetus surrounded by this strength. This is the baby to come. Perhaps this is the feeling of the fourth empty quadrant in the secret garden.

This cave with a lake is like the cave of the womb. It is in the shape of a crescent moon.

The frog indicates a change, movement on many levels.

In Celtic and Welsh mythology, the stag draws the hero into a sacred grove. The stag brings light. In the Middle Ages the people looked to see a light between the antlers. This stag is here to bring some light to the situation. The negative side of the stag is connected with the snake. There is a myth that the stag evokes the snakes out of their holes. The stag breathes in the snake and digests it. As soon as he digests the snake, the antlers change. The snake sheds its skin as a renewal and the stag changes its antlers. The snake is seen as the enemy, the dark side of the stag.

Here the stag comes in from the side. He is not taking part in the scene that is going on in this tray. We will have to see if he brings the light, or whether he is the guide for a holy path, or if he brings up the connection with the snake.

The star stone is standing up this time. Maybe this indicates that something is going to move, like a wheel, especially regarding the birth process.

She had a round lake in the last tray. Here there is a star-shaped configuration with the fish. Maybe this symbol of wholeness has come out of paradise.

The waterfall often comes from a spring in the earth. There is great energy and power in the waterfall. It takes a sudden drop, like the water breaking in the birth.

## Tray 15
## Pregnant Woman

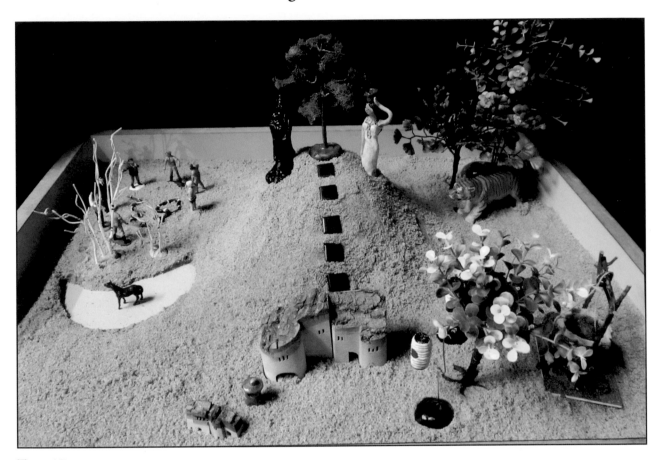

**Tray 15a**
**Pregnant Woman**

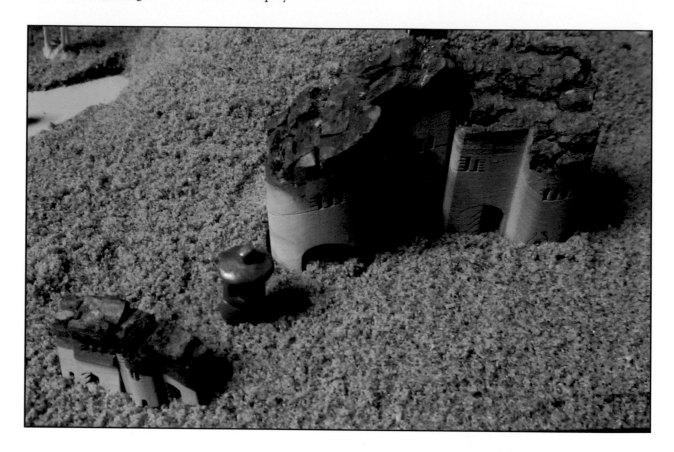

*Her house, near left*

**Tray 15b**
**Pregnant Woman**

*This is the house my father gave me before he died.*

Kwan Yin is the Goddess of Mercy in China and Japan. She is feminine. In India and Tibet it is masculine, or both. This is an all-embracing capacity. She is a Bodhisattva. The Bodhisattva is a follower of Buddha who has promised to not enter into nirvana until all human beings are safe. This indicates a tremendous capacity for compassion.

The Kwan Yin is probably seen as dark and negative, because the whole scene is dominated by dark experiences. She had a house in her home country that was given to her by her father. However, her mother tore it down when she was in Switzerland. So here it has become negative. The Kwan Yin is dark, because she is not sure about the outcome of the birth. She has an inner and an outer threat. After a paradisiacal situation, the dark sides of things come up. She could not see the light of the situation. She could not see anything but the darkness, even though the Kwan Yin was still here.

In Brazil, the black Madonna is Aparecida. She came out of a river in 1717, in the net of fisherman. She wears a blue coat and is the most venerated Madonna in Brazil.

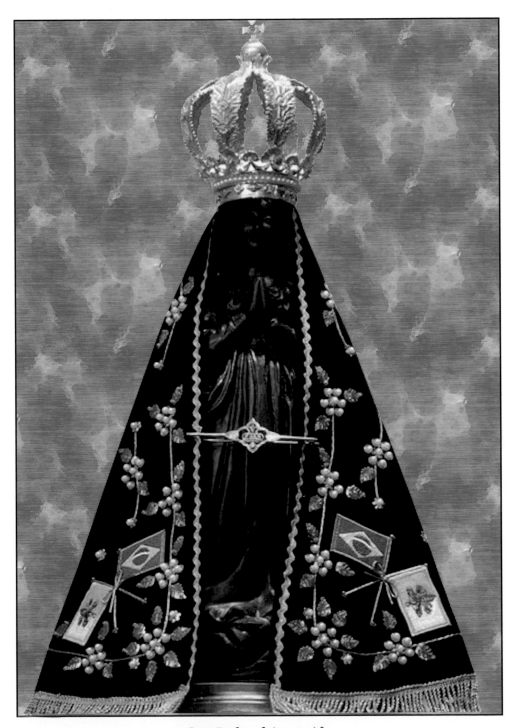

**Our Lady of Aparecida**

Here there are poisonous snakes. The snake played a role in the expulsion from the Garden of Eden. The lake is in the shape of the moon. The small horse in the lake is like the baby in the womb. Also the horse is in danger from snakes. And this is a small horse.

The tiger may be the danger that exists for the woman on the hill. A tiger can spring and attack unpredictably. The tiger is the fierce aspect of the mother. It is aggressive and may be threatening. Kali is carried by a tiger. She is the wrathful aspect of the feminine. Perhaps this shows an aggressive side that she feels she suffers from.

There are seven men. Here we are under the threat of the masculine once again, together with the danger of the little horse. The men here may be her brothers, who were favored over the girls.

The indication of all of these dark experiences may be the beginning of the birth process. Here the shadow comes up. This happens when the mother nears the time of birth. All of the dark animal forces here indicate there may be some suffering. There is danger with anticipating a birth. In the Garden of Eden, God gave women the pain of childbirth. In this tray we can see its darker influences.

## Kali

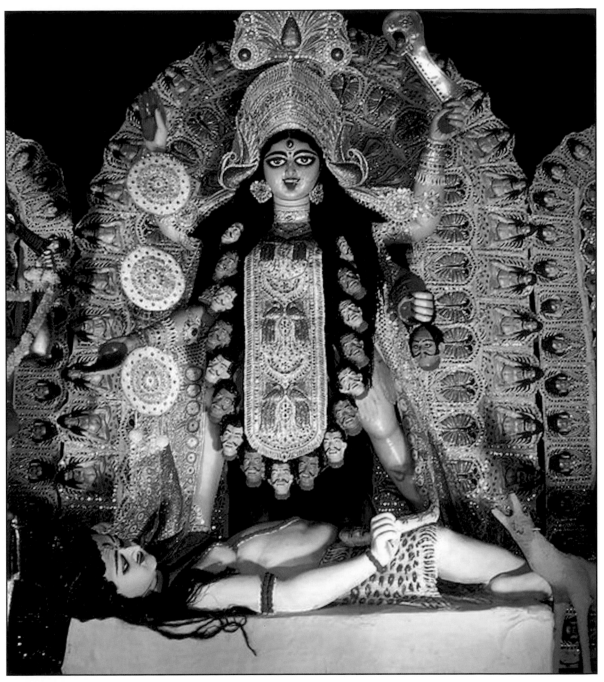

**Kali**
*Photo Jonoikobangali, 2010*

Kali is a ferocious form of the mother goddess, worshipped by Hindus, whose popularity rose with the creation of the *Devi Mahatmya,* a fifth to sixth century religious text. Kali is a complex figure. She is often depicted with four arms, holding a sword and the severed head of a demon in two hands, while her other hands bestow gestures of blessings and dispelling of fear. Her skin is deep blue black and she wears a garland of skulls around her neck.

Kali's name is derived from the Sanskrit word *kala,* which means black or dark colored. This is primarily associated with the dimension of time, indicating that Kali exists prior to the creation of time and space. She is what is beyond time. As the feminine principle, Kali is associated with the god Shiva, the masculine, who represents the round of life and death in creation.

In spite of her fearsome appearance, her devotees have a loving appreciation and reverence for Kali. The classic *Hymn to Kali Karpuradi-Stoti,* translated into English by Arthur Avalon extols Kali's greatness as boundless:

> Oh Mother, even a dullard becomes a poet who meditates upon Thee raimented with space, three-eyed Creatrix of the three worlds, whose waist is beautiful with a girdle made of numbers of dead men's arms, and who on the breast of a corpse, as Thy couch in the cremation-ground, enjoyest Mahakala. (The experience of being unlimited by past, present or future)

Verse 7
*Hymm to Kali Karpuradi-Stotra*

## Tray 16
## Pregnant Woman

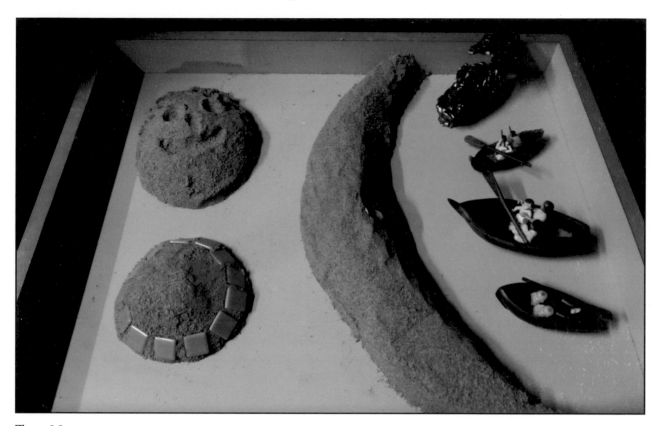

**Tray 16a**
**Pregnant Woman**

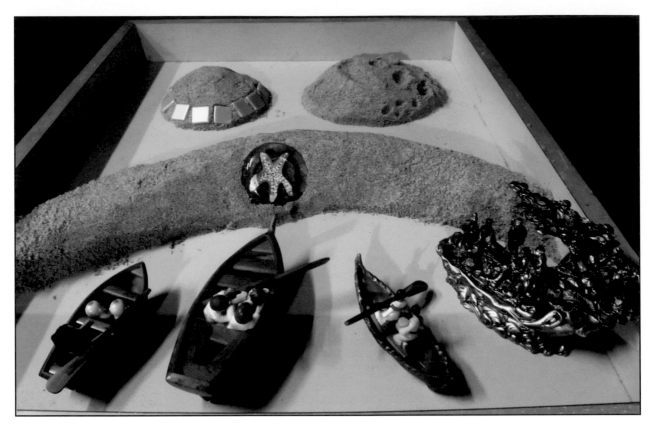

**Tray 16b**
**Pregnant Woman**

Here are the great forces of the coming birth. The star stone is the place to exit, but there is not an opening quite yet. Grof called this a *"No Exit"* situation. The womb is still closed and the child cannot get through. It is like a cervical plug. She is eight and a half months along at this time.

When the child is born, the first things it sees are the eyes and face of the mother. Here is a woman's face and a breast. Perhaps we can see the circle as the breast and the golden stones as the satisfaction of the nourishment it gives.

The boats indicate the pressure of the birth. Perhaps they carry all that the baby comes into the world with – wisdom, nature, etc. The Tibetans say that in the ninth month of pregnancy, the child remembers all of its incarnations. But this is forgotten at the moment of birth. In this respect, the boats could be remembrances.

**Tray 17**
**Pregnant Woman**

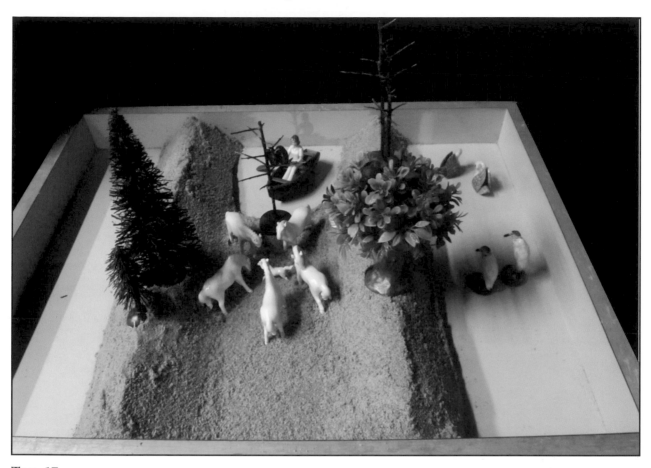

**Tray 17a**
**Pregnant Woman**

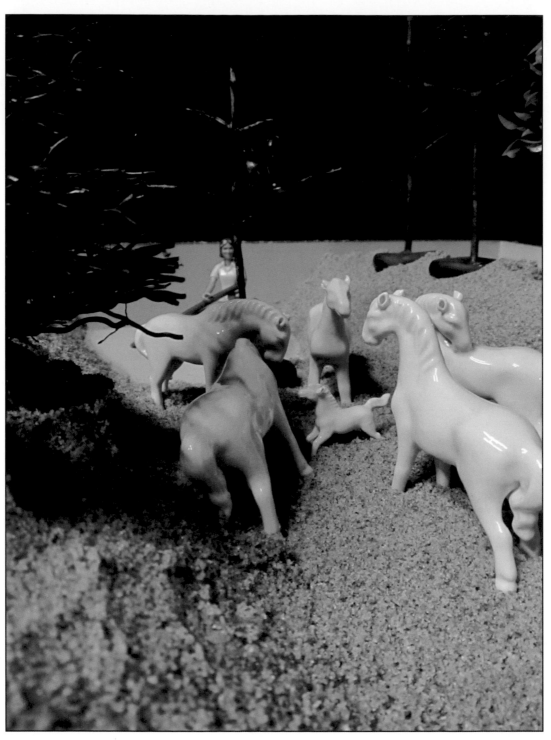

**Tray 17b**
**Pregnant Woman**

She had a dream:

*My mother told me that my sister* (also pregnant) *will die giving birth, and that I will also die.*

This what Grof describes as the third stage of birth, when fear is activated. This came when she had high blood pressure.

This looks like the lower part of the body. Here is the birth. There are two legs and the birth canal with the boat coming out.

The five horses protect the little horse, but he still must pass through the death situation (the ravens) before he gets out. The horses are the forces that protect the child and also the powers that move it. She is showing her will to surrender her body to the process. You must surrender the ego at this moment, or the baby will not come. You cannot watch anymore. You must let go. This is a death of the ego as you know it.

The barren tree is the fear of death. This is felt by many women when they give birth. The swans are a positive side of the birth. In a Greek myth, the swan gives birth to the golden egg of the universe. In the depths of her unconscious, there is hope for a good birth. The barren trees are the barrenness, the aloneness that she feels at this moment, but it will be a beautiful experience afterwards. (The swans) Also, the trees on the left indicate that this is a natural process. The herons are the symbol of long life.

In Hinduism the swan gave birth to a golden ego out of which arose Brahma. (The god of creation) This indicates a positive course for the birth at the same time we see the danger and death in other parts of the tray.

There are two white herons and two black ravens. Here we go from the black to the white again, like the alchemical process. Also she may experience her blackness differently now. After all, the dark ugly duckling becomes the swan.

## Tray 18
## Pregnant Woman

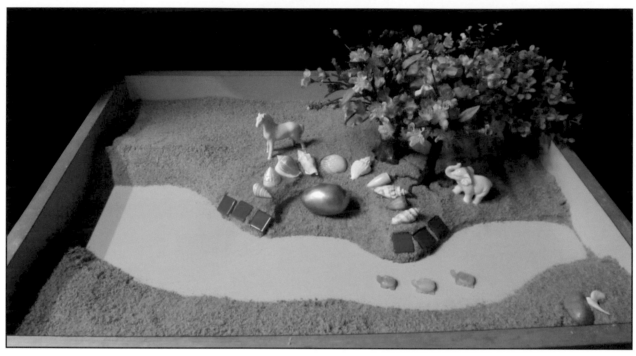

**Tray 18**
**Pregnant Woman**

The golden egg was pre-figured in the last tray. This is the gold egg that Brahma comes out of. Seeing this is a tremendous relief after the struggle of the last tray.

The turtles are a union of opposites. They are a totality of heaven and earth. They have a precious quality and in many mythologies they carry the world. Here it looks as though they come to congratulate the birth.

The white horse and the white elephant carry the sacred quality. This means that the divine is here to help her and to celebrate. There is tremendous relief and thankfulness.

**Tray 19**
**Pregnant Woman**

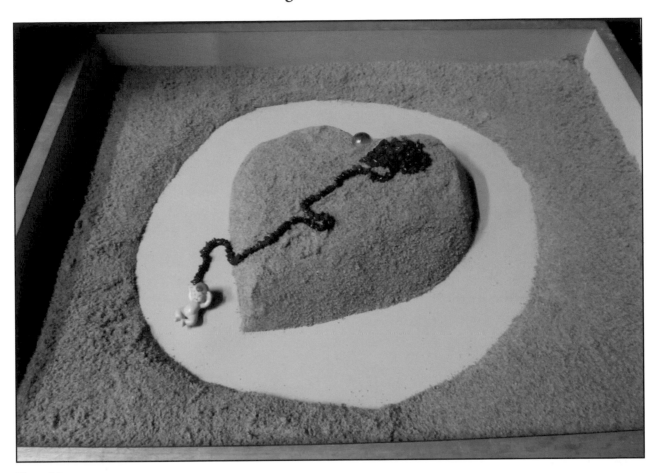

**Tray 19**
**Pregnant Woman**

This is a beautiful image of carrying your baby under your heart. At this time she suffered from high blood pressure.

# Tray 20
# Pregnant Woman

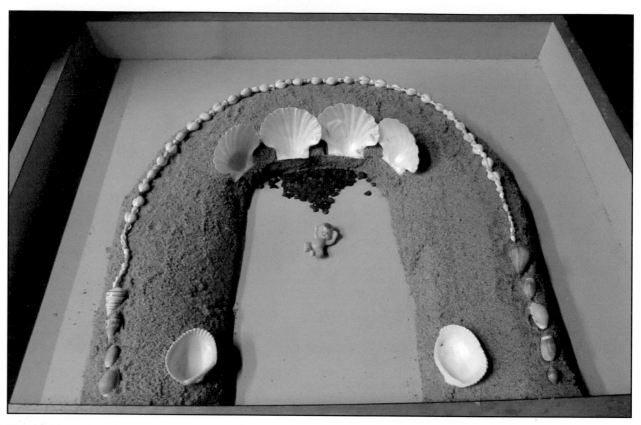

**Tray 20a**
**Pregnant Woman**

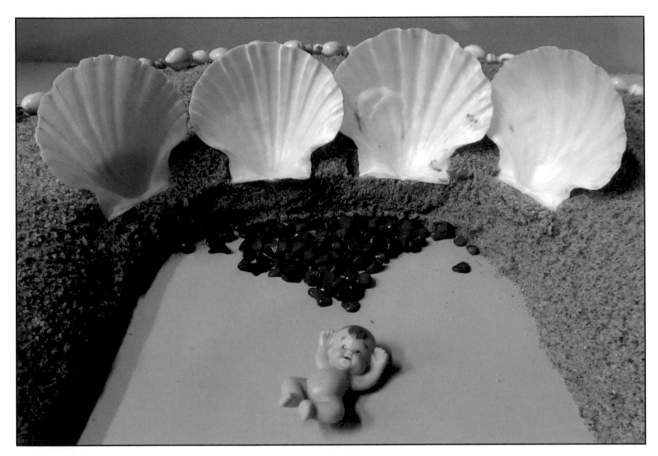

**Tray 20b**
**Pregnant Woman**

This is a picture of birth. Not only is her baby being born, but her inner child is being honored. This was done seven days prior to the birth.

## Tray 21
## Pregnant Woman

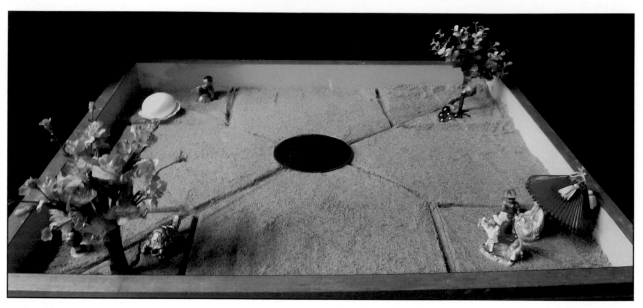

**Tray 21a**
**Pregnant Woman**

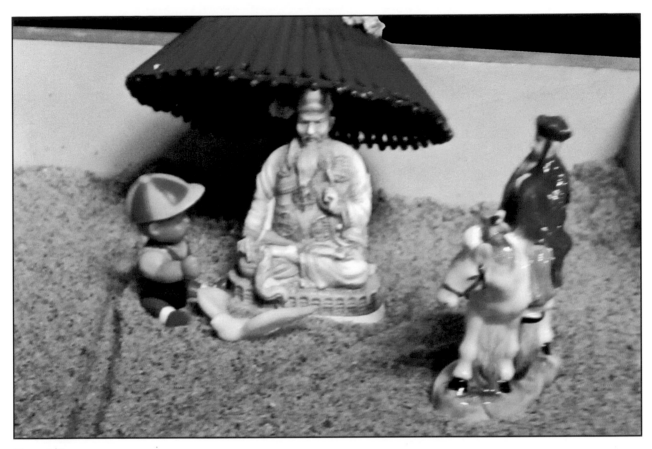

**Tray 21b**
**Pregnant Woman**

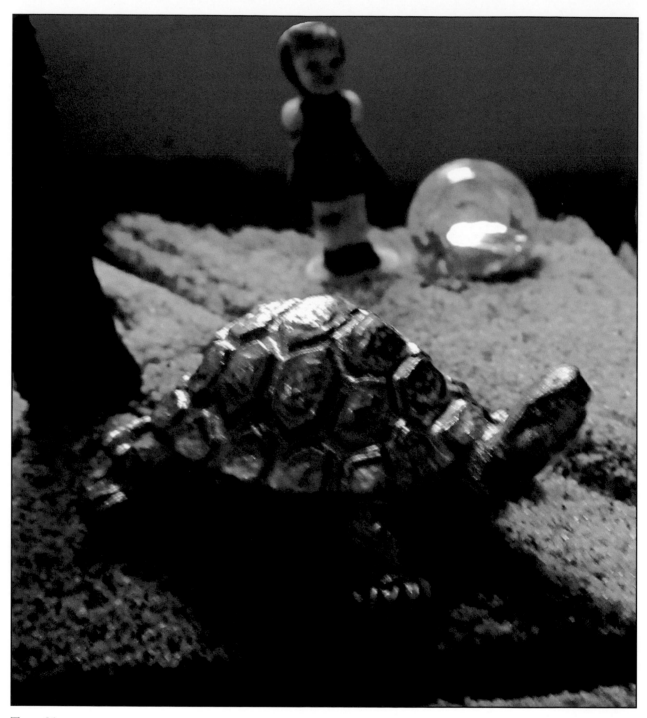

**Tray 21c**
**Pregnant Woman**

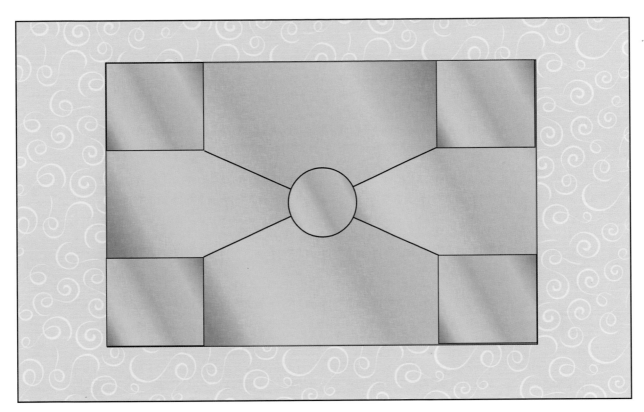

**Tray 21 - Diagram**
**Pregnant Woman**

This was done one day before the birth.

This is like the paradise tray with the mirror in the center, now opening to the four corners of the world. The fourth stage of birth is called *"Inner Peace."* This is a mandala that shows an inner peace. The tray shows that she had already given birth, and it prefigures her inner peace.

The structure of this picture is so different from all of the others. Perhaps there is a concentration that needed to bring order - a waiting for a fulfillment. The empty corner says that it is not yet here. It has a tree with shiny marbles. This is wisdom, or knowledge - the tree of life. That the empty space is next to this indicates maybe a deeper knowledge that is not there, but may come through the birth process. The tension is gone. This is an anticipation of the birth. The trays always show the future situation, not the present situation. This tray foretells the birth. Here there is complete relaxation.

One area is still empty. Perhaps this is her baby that is about to come. In life something new is always coming from the unknown. Here something is due soon.

Here is a man on a white horse. This is a divine vehicle, because the monk who went to China in the time of Buddha to get knowledge is riding on a white horse. He may need to find something precious that aims at inner knowledge.

The red umbrella is protecting the child. In the Far East, the holy men will be protected with an umbrella. This is a protection against all things that could happen.

The man playing the flute is the joy she anticipates. There is an egg in this shell. This is the coming child, the anticipation.

Here there is a golden turtle. In the last picture there were three turtles that came when the golden egg was on the way. Now this is a golden turtle that is very precious.

She scored the sand, connecting each part with the center. She has shaped the circle, the square and the triangle. All is aiming at the central happening. This concentration may be a revelation by the act of birth. The center is very clear and reflects heaven. Remember the cross from the first picture? With the mirror she bears a different cross. This is the Self, the center. It contains everything. She was filled with an inner completeness and confidence.

The baby was born the next day. She had an easy birth. All of my sandplay people tell me they have easy births. Seven days later she came with her new baby girl.

## Tray 22
## Pregnant Woman

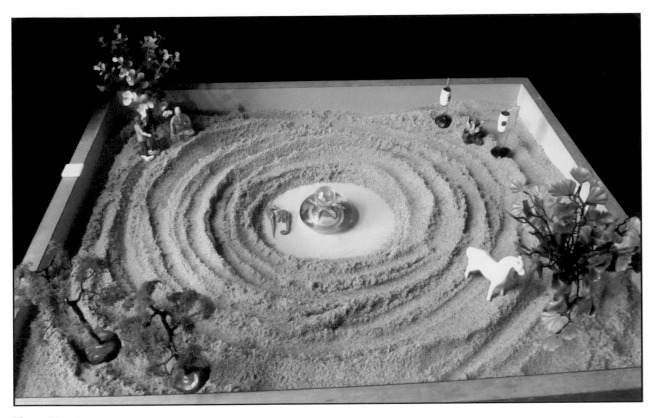

**Tray 22a**
**Pregnant Woman**

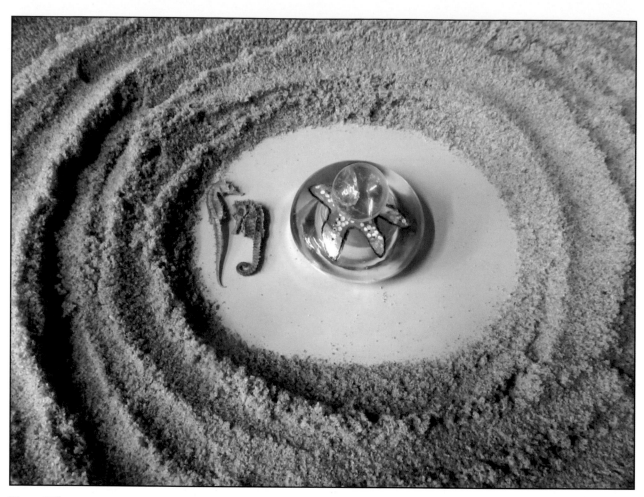

**Tray 22b**
**Pregnant Woman**

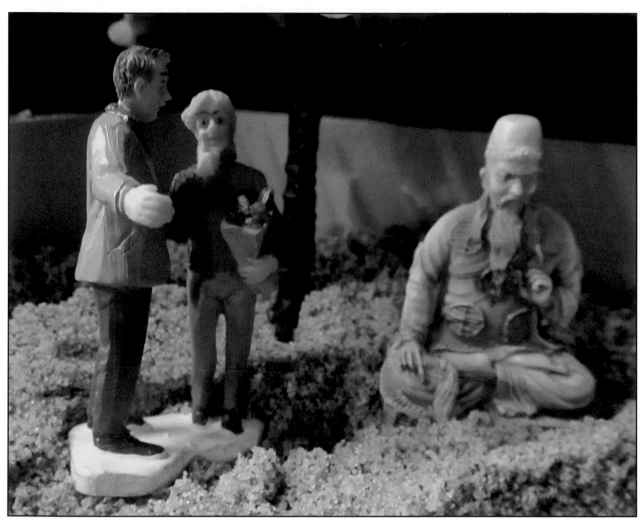

**Tray 22c**
**Pregnant Woman**

This is a whirlpool, like the one she had in the third tray. Here it is tamed. Now the totality is in the center. The star stone and the glass ball have come to the center for the first time. Her sense of Self has come together.

Here are two seahorses. The male seahorse gives birth to the babies. The female lays the eggs in a pouch on the male. If there is danger, the male sucks the babies into his mouth to protect them. This is a very intimate cooperation of the male and female. These animals give birth to their new born children together. They show a unity just like the symbols of wholeness in the center.

Here is a fire that is also illuminated by two lanterns. The fire is light and love. This image is full of fulfillment, harmony and love. The white horse shows the divine quality and an inner gratitude for what has happened.

When we see sequences of images, look to see what is happening by noticing what kind of intentions are coming up. Here the whirlpool indicates a path to the depths. In the third tray with the whirlpool we could not see what was in it. Here it has opened and we can see what it is she is looking for. She called her baby *Pearl*. Maybe through giving birth to her Pearl, she gave birth to her inner pearl. It is a grain of sand that is at the center of the pearl. It is created by irritating the oyster.

There is a little yellow tile on the edge. I do not think she put it there. It was just there.

The integration of the Self is just the beginning. It is never an ending. This is the moment where new life begins. This is the basis for a new beginning. It is just after the constellation of the Self that new life can begin from a very deep level in the person. Often we will see images of nature and animals. This is the instinctual level. This begins an adaptation to daily life.

Now she is ready to deal with the integration of black and white. Until now she had been dealing with giving birth to this baby.

## Tray 23
## Pregnant Woman

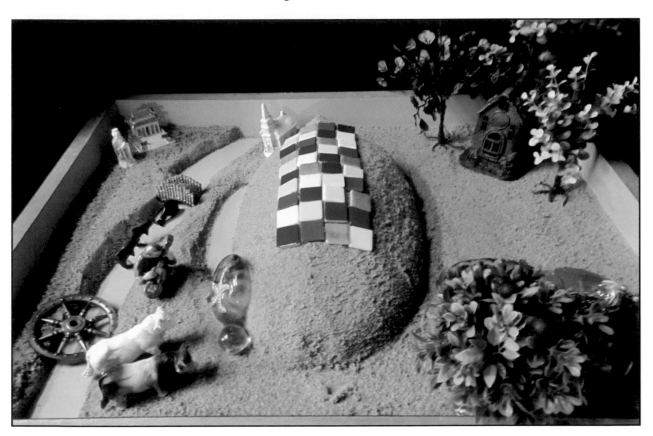

**Tray 23a**
**Pregnant Woman**

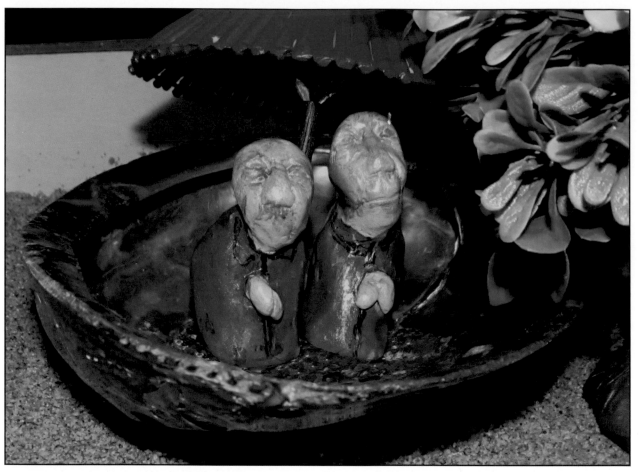

**Tray 23b**
**Pregnant Woman**

The Self is a part of the integration. In Jung's psychology, the individuation process is for the second half of life. It is about becoming more conscious of our journey. When the Self appears for the first time, this is not the Self that we can become conscious of. This is a basis for a new personality to build upon. This will consist of qualities and aspects of the personality that were hidden and unavailable to us, as they were in the unconscious. This is the preliminary Self, as given by birth. This contains a nucleus, a germ of the path to follow. Through our cultural influences we deviate from this path. Through sandplay we penetrate to the depths of our being and have the chance to live more fully. Perhaps then, we can reach that point of which Jung spoke and become more conscious of our journey.

This is an eight-spoke wheel. When Buddha was enlightened it was said that the eight-spoke wheel began to turn. This is the eight-fold path. His wisdom begins to move. We see here that things keep moving, turning. Now it is touching the water. This means it will be turned by the deeper forces of the unconscious.

Here the mound is like another pregnant belly, a womb. It is flame-shaped. It is an alchemical process. There are two bulls in front of the star stone and the "pearl." The man and the bulls approach the star stone with instinctual nature. In Greek mythology, bulls are sacrificed before a birth. This may indicate that a new birth is taking place. This pregnant belly is full of all of these colors. The color tiles are Jung's four personality types. This also indicates a new beginning.

Here the star stone leans against the wall of the belly. It is like the exit to the full belly we saw before. This time the little pearl is already outside of the belly. But something else is going to be born. The bulls wait at the door.

Here is an elderly couple under the umbrella in a shell. When older people appear in dreams, we feel that these are situations we have to change. Here they stand in a shell where something can come forth. Maybe this is a renewal of an old situation. The apple tree carries the fruit of transformation.

We also see three dolphins. When a dolphin gives birth, three others come to midwife. Here they come to assist with the transformation.

Here is a Christian church and a Chinese temple and a wise man with a bridge between them. The Chinese philosophy is connected with deeper realms and with nature, whereas this is missing in the Christian Church. They come together now.

## Tray 24
## Pregnant Woman

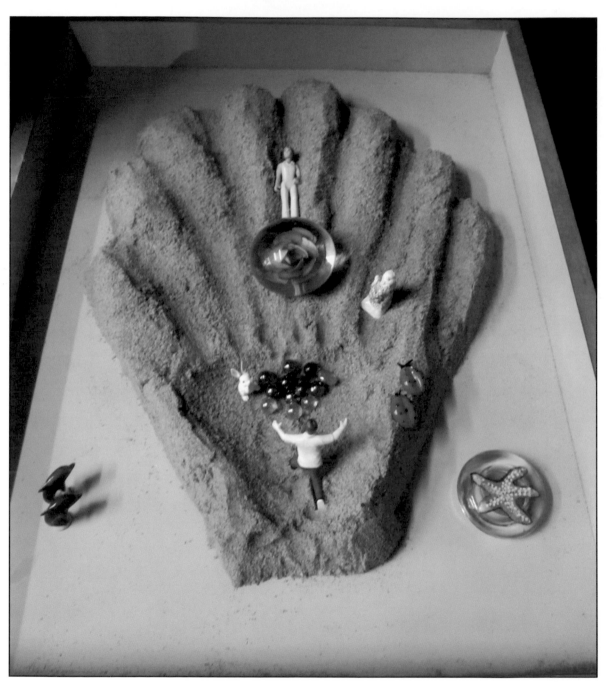

**Tray 24**
**Pregnant Woman**

Here is another birth. This is a birth to her worldly self. The sand looks like a shell. Here a white woman is born into God's hands. This is the birth of her valuing herself with the same values as a white woman.

This is the birth of herself as "white," seeing herself as of equal value. Now she can accept herself as a dark-skinned woman with a full value. She can break through to this wholeness after the picture of the birth.

Never stop at the point of the Self. We see that this is her new beginning. When the Self is constellated, the Self is very tender. It must be protected.

Erich Neumann talked of stages of (ego) development: (Following the constellation of the Self)

1. Animal – Vegetative level
2. Fighting Stage – Horse stage for girls - This is the discussion with the world
3. Adaptation to the Collective - Integration

Maybe the renewal of the feminine qualities is more important for the girls, so they become acquainted with the world - thus the horses.

This birth is in a shell, like the birth of Venus. Also it is like being carried in God's hand. The man with open arms receives her with joy and reverence. This is also the shape of an inverted triangle, the feminine. Before the marbles were in the triangle with the tree, next to the empty space. Perhaps this empty space is this new acceptance of herself.

The ladybugs are good luck. They are a happy sign.

The sea star is on the sea stone. This is a sign of fulfillment, as there are the five elements coming together: Earth – yellow; water – white; fire – red; air – green; and spirit – blue.

Here is a lotus flower. Now she shows the feminine qualities in the form of the flower. In the Far East the lotus is a symbol of the totality of the Self.

In the last picture we saw dolphins swimming toward the Christian church and the Chinese temple. They remind us of the union of the two sides of religion, the integration of the intellectual and the more natural.

The rabbit is a feminine symbol. In early Christianity the fox and the rabbit were good friends. The monks could not talk about women, so took the symbol of the rabbit. By the beginning of the thirteenth century, the fox was killing the rabbit. This was the beginning of the supremacy of the intellect over the feminine quality. In the East the fox and the hare remained good friends. The Chinese say, *"When the hare dies, the fox cries."*

We are living in a time when the feminine is trying to emerge again. But we are not doing this in the best way. We put too much emphasis on the intellect. The best feminine qualities are compassion, being able to carry, to support.

---

## Participant Question

*What would you advise about the use of sandplay with psychotic patients?*

Sandplay can be very healing after a psychotic episode, but not before. A researcher in Japan found it very helpful to paint a dark border around the paper the psychotic patients used for their art work. Professor Kawai said he would not do sandplay with someone who began by putting a line of fencing up against the edge of the tray, as they had psychotic tendencies. If they draw with their fingers around the tray, this is a warning of psychosis, also.

Clients who fill the trays very full may be afraid of the free space. They may be afraid that the deeper materials may surface.

---

**Tray 25**
**Pregnant Woman**

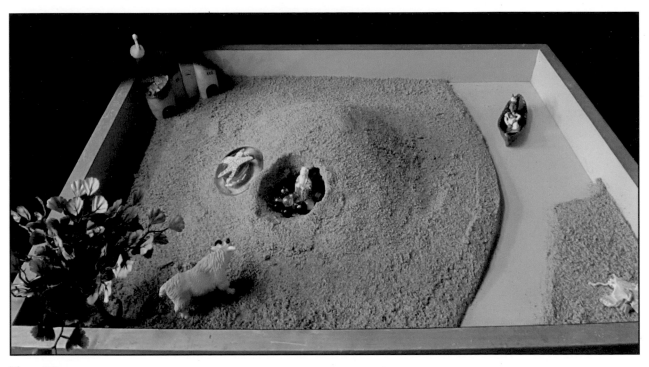

**Tray 25a**
**Pregnant Woman**

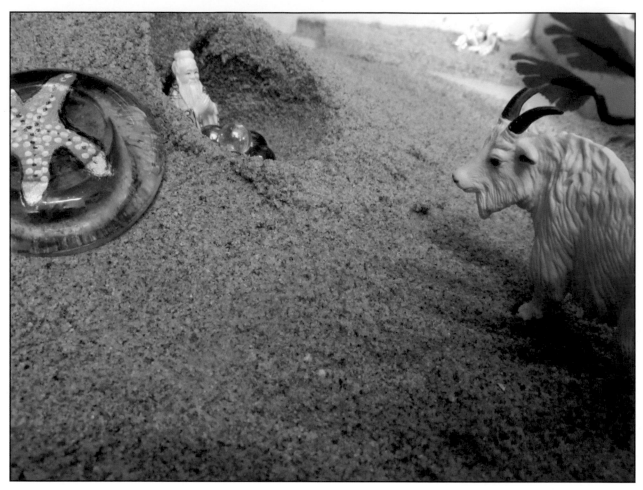

**Tray 25b**
**Pregnant Woman**

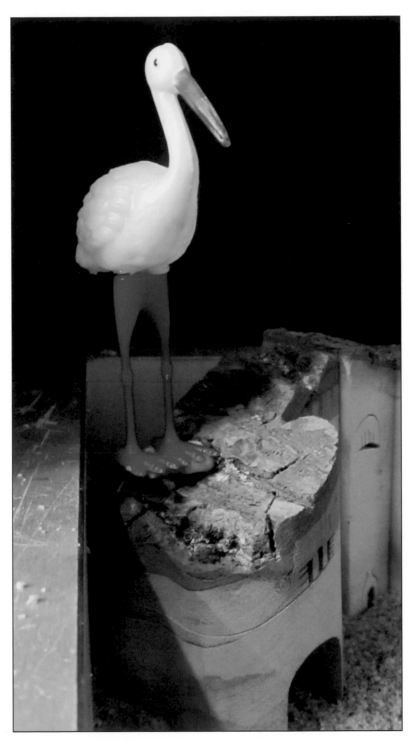

**Tray 25c**
**Pregnant Woman**

This is now a third birth - to the spirit itself. First there was her real baby. Then the dark woman was reborn with the value of white. And now we have the birth of the spiritual life.

She said this was like the cave opening to Jesus. This puts her fully in tune with her environment and she is having a spiritual experience.

The stork brings the children from heaven down to earth. The mountain goat can climb very high in the mountains. They are sure-footed on steep places. This is a spiritual animal that can commune with God in the high places. The goat is also a very sexual animal.

The little house is like the one that her father gave her, but her mother had it taken away.

## Tray 26
## Pregnant Woman

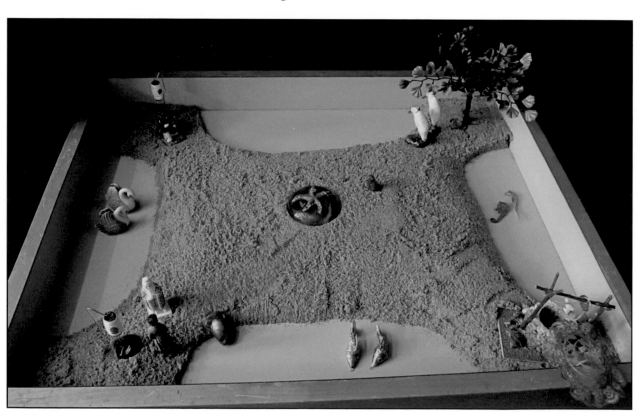

**Tray 26a**
**Pregnant Woman**

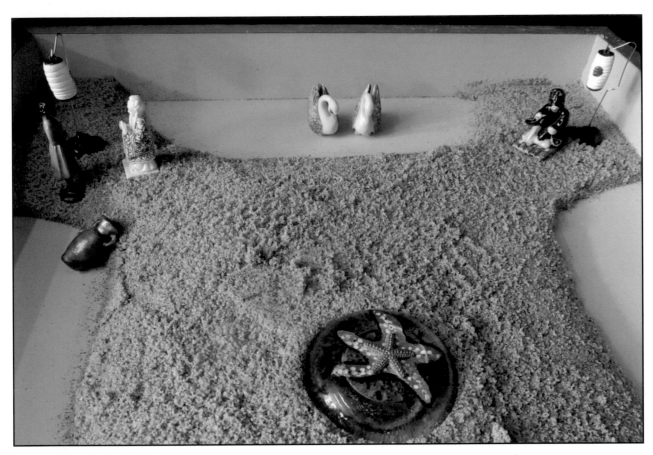

**Tray 26b**
**Pregnant Woman**

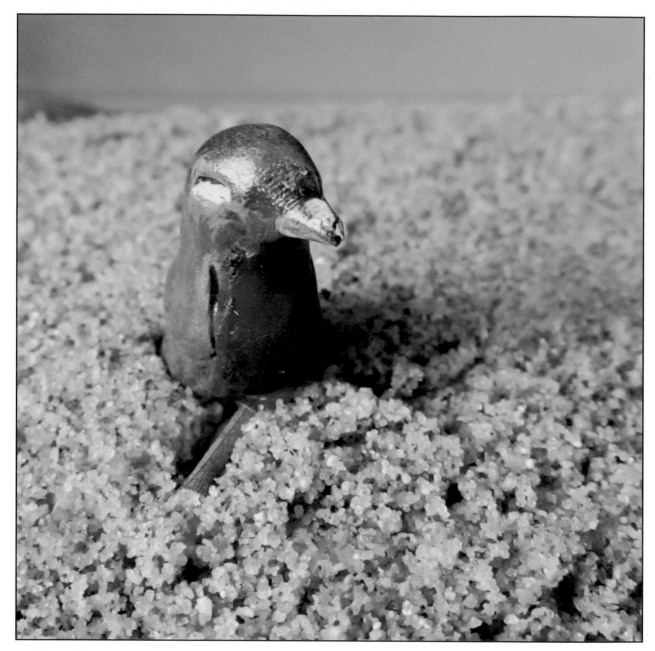

**Tray 26c**
**Pregnant Woman**

The robin is the first bird of Spring. The robin gave Jesus something to drink when he was on the cross. His breast touched the blood of Christ and has been red ever since. The robin has a good relationship with people. He tried to pull the thorns from Christ's body and covered his body with leaves. Here we see her intimate relationship to the religious quality. Her relationship to Christianity begins to transform. The problems that surfaced in the beginning are developing into their opposites. This takes place after the centering of the Self. The robin is a healing agent for the Christ. Here it is a healing of the Christianity.

Herons and swans can go into the water and they can fly. Seahorses and fish stay in the water. These are gold fish and are of great value. This is the Christ. The swans are the union of opposites, as are the seahorses. Here we cover the water, land and air, the various levels of the personality.

Here is a jar, a vessel, or amphora. Amphorae were used in the Middle Ages and in Rome as containers for wine. Many were lost on the journeys across the sea and are found at the bottom of the sea. Perhaps she has found a feminine side from the depths of the unconscious and is making its presence known on the earth. There is also a well where we get more contents from the very depths.

This picture covers the four corners of the world. There is an opening to new dimensions.

The blue umbrella is a protector. This time it is a parasol. Perhaps it was a protection against too much light, or going too fast.

## Tray 27
## Pregnant Woman

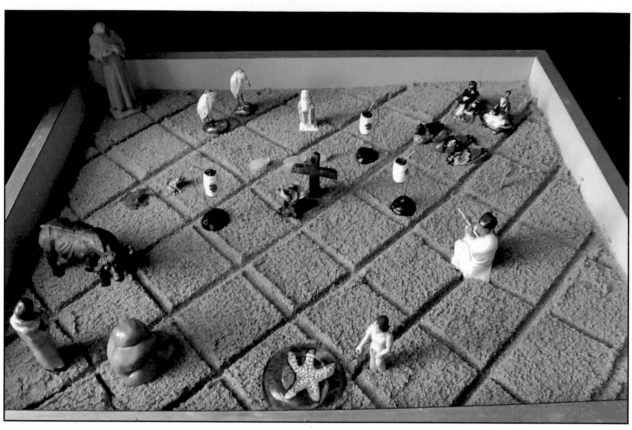

**Tray 27a**
**Pregnant Woman**

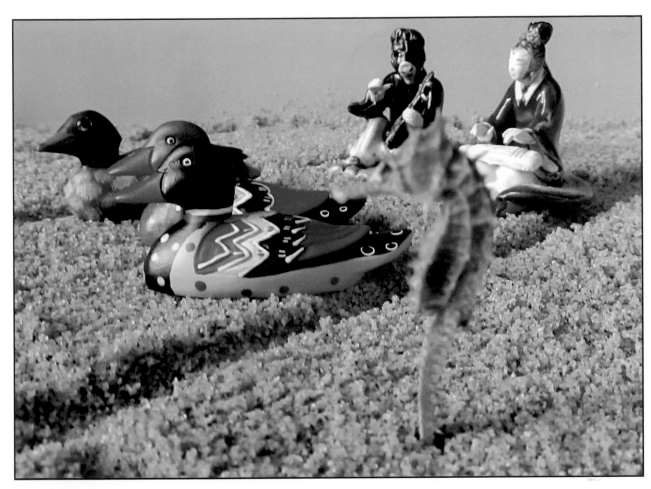

**Tray 27b**
**Pregnant Woman**

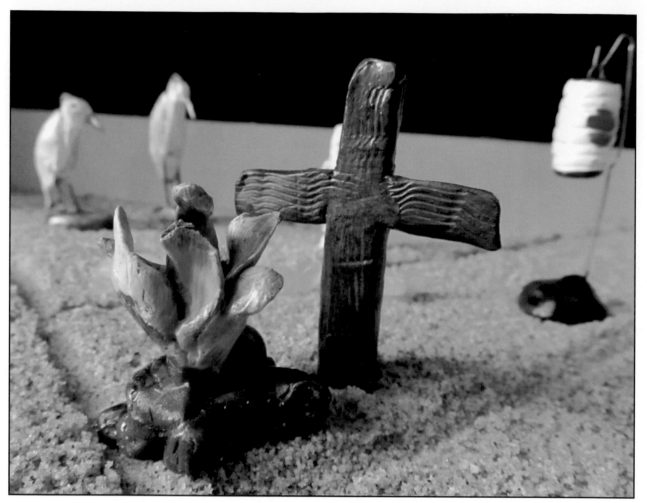

**Tray 27c**
**Pregnant Woman**

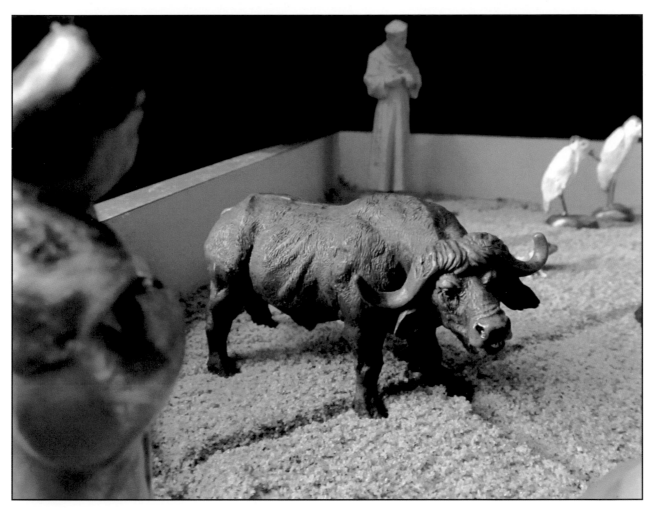

**Tray 27d**
**Pregnant Woman**

The shapes in the sand are like the cuts of a diamond. Grof commented that this is, "*...a diamond with many facets.*" This feels very strong. This brings together everything that has been important during her process. The fire and the cross now come together in the center. At the beginning she hung upside down between two crosses. Now the love and the cross are brought together.

The Chinese women are devoted to their music, to love and feeling. The lanterns are like those used in a temple area, a holy place. The man with the flute is a new animus in contrast with the pondering man.

The ox may indicate that the mind needs to be tamed in order to become enlightened. In the sand the mind, the body and the spirit work together. All three factors have a part in it.

St. Francis was a wealthy man who left everything behind and lived in a little hut. He was able to talk with the animals. He understood nature and the animal world. This is what she was learning – that religion cannot just be known through the head, but must be known through the instincts. St. Francis appears where the Chinese temple and the Christian church were previously.

The facets of the diamond are part of the whole. They all work together. They also look like the fields of the earth. They contain the parts of herself that she values.

## Tray 28
## Pregnant Woman

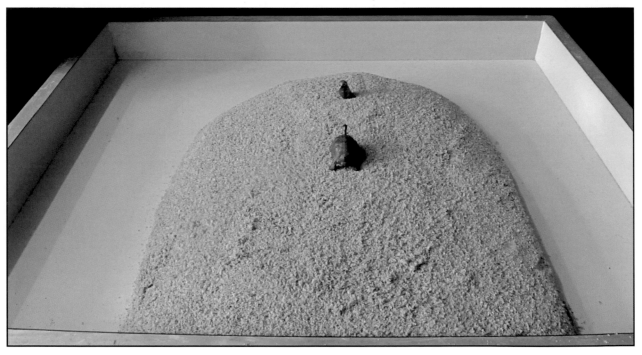

**Tray 28a**
**Pregnant Woman**

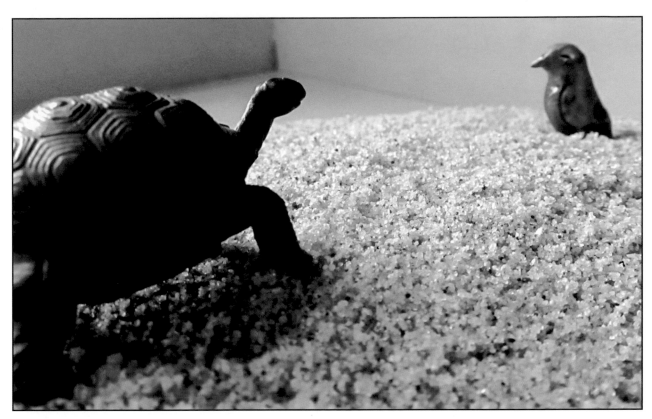

**Tray 28b**
**Pregnant Woman**

This is a symbol of heaven and earth - the robin and the turtle. Here they are on another womb, telling us that she has these qualities that complete herself. She said the robin and the turtle are talking to each other. The earth and the sky come together. She did many similar trays between this one and the final tray.

**Tray 29**
**Pregnant Woman**
**Final Tray**

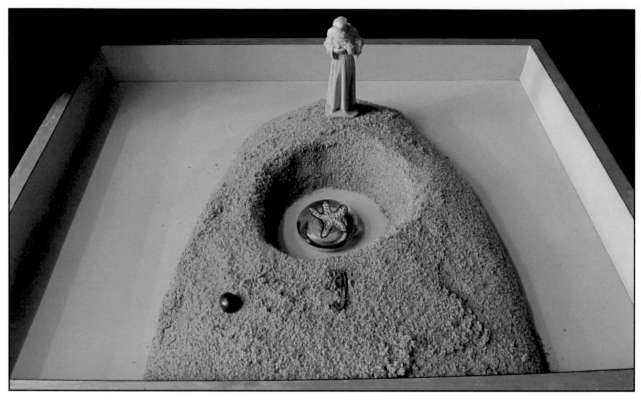

**Tray 29a**
**Pregnant Woman**

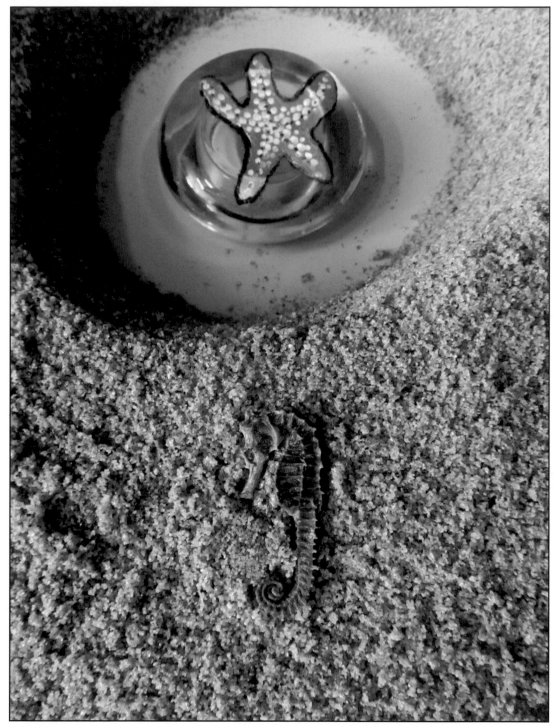

**Tray 29b**
**Pregnant Woman**

This is an image that goes beyond our verbal reality. It is more abstract. St. Francis becomes more important to her. The star stone is shown to have great value. This shows the value of living together with the instinctual life and the religious way.

The seahorse combines the masculine and the feminine in itself. We must use both sides of the personality, the balance of the masculine and the feminine.

She was leaving soon after this and was perhaps a little afraid of returning to her native country. Maybe she needed the strength from religion to carry her through. This was a great problem to her in the beginning. Now this may be her security to undertake new things.

This entire process took just about one year. The wise man usually talks very little. Perhaps this is why these latter trays are so simple.

---

## Participant Questions

*Do you make an interpretation as a closure with the client?*

We usually do not make any interpretation for a closure. If you undergo the process, you do not have to say much, because you feel it. To interpret would disturb or stop the process. To interpret is a big mistake. You must have the courage to let the process happen, to trust that it will happen in the right way.

*Is sandplay suitable for autistic children?*

Many children that are called autistic are not actually that. Often they are very withdrawn, but are very talented. Many are quite musical. They are highly sensitive. You must treat them carefully. Truly autistic children would be very hard to work with in the sand. See how they respond. One such child only wanted to hear songs that had to do with the night and the moon. Very slowly he changed, but it took a long time. He would sit on my knees, as I played the piano and sang to him.

*Do you often use music in your work with sandplay?*

I sometimes use music. When young children hear jazz or rock they make disturbed designs in the tray. When I play Bach, their designs come into place. It has a very good influence on them. I need to work toward an inner peace, so what has been thwarted can come up. I use music to bring them to the center.

*What is happening when children put things in and take them out of the tray, and move them around a lot?*

When this happens there is some inner disturbance. It shows that they cannot concentrate. You must work to contain their experience. When you can do this, they will calm down. When this is going on I must concentrate all the more. This gives the security they need.

*What do you do when children want to use two trays?*

I will let them do it, but I know that they cannot concentrate on what they are doing.

---

**End**
**Pregnant Woman**

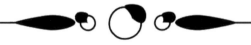

# References Mentioned in Text

Avalon, A. (1922). *Hymn to Kali karpuradi-stotra.* London: Luzac & Co.

Cheng'en, W. (1999). *Journey to the west.* (W.J.F. Jenner, Trans.) Beijing: Foreign Languages Press. (Original 16th c.)

Goethe, J.W. (2010). *Reineke fox, west-eastern divan, and achilleid.* (A. Rogers, Trans.) Charleston, SC: Nabu Press. (Original work published 1890)

Grof, S. (1996). *Realms of the human unconscious: Observations from LSD research.* London: Souvenir Press Ltd. (Original work published 1976)

Grof, S. (1984). *Ancient wisdom and modern science.* New York: State University of New York.

Grof, S. (1985). *Beyond the brain: birth, death, and transcendence in psychotherapy.* New York: State University of New York.

Grof, S. (1988). *The adventure of self-discovery: Dimensions of consciousness and new perspectives in psychotherapy and inner exploration.* New York: State University of New York.

Grof, S. (1989). *Spiritual emergency: when personal transformation becomes a crisis.* New York: Tarcher.

Jung, C.G. (1968). *Aion: Researches into the phenomenology of the self.* (R.F.C. Hull, Trans.) Princeton: Princeton University Press. (Original work published 1959)

Jung, C.G. (1977). *Psychology and alchemy.* (R.F.C. Hull, Trans.) Princeton: Princeton University Press. (Original work published 1953)

Kalff, D. (1957). The significance of the hare in Renard the Fox. *Journal of Analytical Psychology 2* (2), 183–193.

Neumann, E. (1995). *Origins and history of consciousness.* Princeton: Princeton University Press. (Original work published 1954)

Saint-Exupery, A. (1995). *The little prince.* Hertfordshire: Wordsworth Editions Limited. (Original work published 1971)

Schiller, F.C. (2010). *Poems of the Third Period.* Charleston, SC: BiblioBazaar. (Original work published 18th c.)

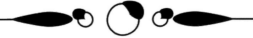

# Resources for Sandplay Training

International Society for Sandplay Therapy – ISST
www.isst-society.com

Sandplay Therapists of America – STA
www.sandplay.org

Barbara Turner, PhD
*International Training Programs in Sandplay*
Certified Sandplay Therapist – Teacher
Registered Play Therapist – Supervisor
www.barbaraturner.org
publisher@temenospress.com

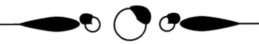

# About the Editor

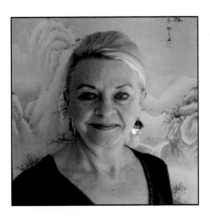

**Barbara A. Turner** is an internationally recognized teacher of Jungian sandplay therapy, as taught by Dora M. Kalff. She offers training programs around the globe. Dr. Turner is the author of *The Handbook of Sandplay Therapy* and co-author with Dr. Kristín Unnsteinsdóttir of *Sandplay and Storytelling: The Impact of Imaginative Thinking on Children's Learning and Development.* In addition, Dr. Turner edited and returned to print the classic works in sandplay: Dora M. Kalff's, *Sandplay: A Psychotherapeutic Approach to the Psyche;* Estelle L. Weinrib's, *Images of the Self: The Sandplay Therapy Process;* and *H.G. Wells' Floor Games: A Father's Account of Play and Its Legacy of Healing.* She lives in Northern California with her husband, author and educator, Thomas Armstrong, PhD.

Dr. Turner is passionate about the profound healing and transformational possibilities inherent in sandplay therapy and is honored to share these materials with you. She welcomes your comments and feedback.

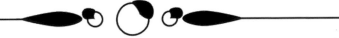

# Index

## A

*absolution*, 28

*abuse*, 132

Acupuncture, 187

aggressive, 1, 11, 78, 82, 278

*Aion*, 240

air, 34, 37, 43, 52, 90, 188, 189, 250, 303, 311

*albedo*, 229

alchemical, 204, 285, 301

alchemy, 229, 234

alligator, 11

American, 173, 177, 207

amphora, 311

analyst, 27, 56, 261

androgynous, 155

animal, 13, 23, 36, 39, 68, 131, 142, 152, 192, 199, 204, 205, 208, 240, 271, 278, 308, 316

animals, 8, 27, 29, 36, 37, 39, 40, 52, 85, 99, 111, 130, 131, 152, 170, 203, 204, 239, 240, 297, 298, 316

animal-vegetative, 13, 23, 68, 159, 193, 204, 205, 208

animus, 121, 157, 173, 174, 176, 183, 185, 208, 217, 218, 247, 315

annunciation, 243

antler(s), 274

Aparecida, 277

apocalypse, 78, 112

apple, 131, 301

Arabs, 114

archetype, 1, 11, 23, 105, 195

art, 78, 155, 304

Arthur Waley, 113

artist, 155

artistic, 14, 23, 49, 61, 81, 209, 218

attitude, 17, 44, 48, 52, 108, 152, 189, 199, 230, 273

*autistic*, 320

autumn, 234

Avalon, Arthur, 280

Ayurvedic, 187

Aztecs, 176, 260

## B

*Ba*, 124

babies, 257, 260, 267, 297, *See* baby

baby, 1, 27, 78, 115, 230, 240, 247, 249, 261, 270, 271, 274, 278, 282, 285, 287, 289, 294, 298, 308

Bach, 320

baptism, 124, 145

baptized, 128, 204

barber, 175, 176

barren, 7, 33, 78, 239, 285

battle, 24, 47, 49

bear, 27

Bear 28

Bellyn, 29, 30

Bible, 128

birth, vii, 1, 2, 12, 43, 56, 61, 71, 104, 115, 118, 137, 166, 192, 203, 206, 219, 229, 239, 243, 249, 255, 257, 261, 263, 271, 273, 274, 276, 278, 282, 285, 286, 289, 293, 294, 297, 298, 300, 301, 303, 308

black, 36, 58, 145, 176, 192, 194, 195, 200, 232, 235, 255, 257, 260, 267, 277, 280, 285, 298

bleeding, 180

blood, 180, 206, 246, 285, 287, 310

blue, 42, 122, 195, 234, 243, 254, 273, 277, 280, 303, 311

Blue, 24, 43, 234

boat, 11, 91, 285

## U

## V

## W